Healing Wounded Doctor-Patient Relationships

"Packed with information that anyone who ever goes to a doctor for any reason deserves to know and that every professional who wants to maximize his or her healing power must understand."

—Tamara Schimke, R.N. and patient

"A giant step closer to the ideal of a fully communicating medical team. This book strips away the clutter and leads doctor and patient directly to the real issues."

—Thomas R. McElderry, M.D.

"This book is beautifully written! I appreciated your attempt to treat both doctors and patients with dignity. It is <u>very</u> well done!"

—Mary L. Ezzo, M.D.

"Outstanding resource for patients and doctors alike. No one who reads this book will walk away without tools to incorporate change in the doctor-patient relationship."

—Sefra Pitzele, author of *We Are Not Alone: Learning to Live With Chronic Illness* (Workman Publishing)

"The topic is very relevant and the book is important . . . As I found in teaching communication, the patient's perspective is invaluable to the physician and a strong addition to the objective data presented in most research in this field."

—John C. Butler, M.D.

"This book is a valuable resource. I learned a great deal from reading it."

—Gregory L. Silvis, M.D.

Healing Wounded Doctor-Patient Relationships

Linda Hanner

with contributions by
John J. Witek, M.D.

KASHAN PUBLISHING

Edited by: Carol J. Frick

Cover and book design by: BookTech

Published by: Kashan Publishing
P.O. Box 307
Delano, MN 55328

© 1995 Linda Hanner

Publisher's Cataloging-in-Publication Data

Hanner, Linda
Healing Wounded Doctor-Patient Relationships/by Linda Hanner
Includes bibliographical references and index.
ISBN 0-9622669-3-0: $14.95
1. Physician and patient.   2. Patient education.
3. Medical consultation.   4. Medicine—Popular.
5. Self care—Health.   I. Title
1995   LCCN: 95-94333

To my husband, Kim, for his patience, once again, during the countless evening and weekend hours I have spent buried in this lengthy project and for lending an ear in my absence to people who call after reading my other books to share their own medical woes.

Some names of patients have been changed to protect their privacy.

FOREWORD

W E HAVE dramatic new tools for diagnosis and treatment of almost every disorder and yet the foundation of medical care—the doctor-patient relationship—is itself in need of diagnosis and treatment!

The relationship is in a state of change. No single physician can provide every medical service for diagnosis and treatment, which puts increasing responsibility on patients themselves to make decisions. They need to be able to communicate with their doctors if they are to learn to navigate the complicated health care system of the late 20th century. The quality of the relationships patients have with their doctors can have significant impact on their health care experience. At the same time, ever increasing demands on physicians for documentation and cost control have erected numerous barriers in the traditional doctor-patient relationship.

This book should be assigned reading for all health care students and providers, as well as for patients, particularly those with chronic or incompletely diagnosed conditions. Linda Hanner has personal experience as a patient and has interviewed many physicians and patients in preparation for writing on this subject. She offers a positive perspective on understanding and improving the doctor-patient relationship.

In a well balanced presentation, not only are the top 10 complaints that patients have about physicians examined, but also the top 10 things that drive physicians crazy in the modern health care system. No great societal change or health care plan is needed for individual patients and doctors to benefit from this book as they seek to decrease the hassles and improve the satisfaction in dealing with medical issues.

A common symptom such as "chest pain" may be a minor chest wall pain or a sign of an impending major heart attack. It may be related to "heartburn" from gastroesophageal reflux, mitral valve prolapse, inflammation (pericarditis), or significant narrowing of one or more coronary arteries—to name a few of the possible causes of this common symptom. Working through the diagnosis and treatment of a common problem such as chest pain—and many other problems— requires doctor and patient to work together as a team.

Where there is technology there can still be appropriate touch and caring, and where there are unsolved illnesses there can still be compassion and communication and appropriate use of referral and other resources. Where there are interfering third parties, there can also be appropriate communication along with a sense of humor. Where there is a chronic or incurable condition, there can still be hope and support to live in what William Osler called "day tight compartments."

The doctor-patient relationship is wounded but not mortally ill. Individual doctors and patients can make a difference in each other's lives through mutual respect and caring, and appropriate use of health care resources. This is the challenge for each of us, and this book contributes greatly to the understanding and management of wounded doctor-patient relationships.

—Stephen R. Yarnall, M.D.
Stevens Cardiology Group, Edmonds, Washington,
Clinical Assoc. Prof. of Medicine, Univ. of Washington,
contributing editor and columnist, HOPE HEALTHLETTER,
author of THE NEW DR. COOKIE COOKBOOK

ACKNOWLEDGMENTS

Once again, it was the willingness of so many others to share their stories that has made this book possible. There are too many to mention, but I want to thank everyone who has been involved for believing in this project enough to be a part of it.

PREFACE

This book, *Healing Wounded Doctor-Patient Relationships*, is the third book borne of my experience with a long undiagnosed illness. The first was a personal account of my search for a diagnosis. More than six years after its publication, calls and letters continue to reinforce that it wasn't just my story, but was representative of the struggles of countless others. The second book, a "self-help" book for people with undiagnosed illness, was forming in my mind as I labored at the first. I knew the book was needed as I became increasingly aware of the misconceptions that most lay people have of the diagnostic process and medical science in general.

I believe the topic of this third book is also immensely important. During the writing of it, I was continually inspired by each visit to a patient support group or chat with a physician. Whenever and wherever I discussed my book and the issues I planned to address, I was met with enthusiasm from doctors and patients alike—*they* believed that it needed to be written and it was with their encouragement that I continued.

This book is based on seven years of research into the evolution and current state of the doctor-patient relationship and interviews with doctors and patients around the nation. Through my research and personal experience, I've learned how the doctor-patient relationship has been set up to fail over time, and why much advice and teaching offered by modern patient advocates and medical trainers has more than likely contributed to the animosity between patients and doctors. Thousands of interviews with patients and dozens with physicians have reinforced what many studies have also shown—patients are angry at doctors for not living up to their expectations, and doctors are defensive and disillusioned by patient mistrust and by the difficulties they face in practicing medicine the way they feel it should be practiced.

This book is based on the premise that there is hope for reconciliation in the doctor-patient rift. It is possible to develop healthy relationships that are healing for patients and rewarding for doctors. I wouldn't have believed that so strongly if it hadn't been for the relationship that I had with Dr. John Witek during the last few years of my own illness. One of the reasons I asked John to work closely with me on the writing of this book was that I realized he had developed a way of working with patients that others could learn a great deal from. I hoped to capture the essence of his style as well as that of other physicians who have a reputation for developing a good rapport with patients. As John and I worked on this project and others, we haven't always agreed on every aspect of every issue. It has taken patience and a willingness to be open to each other's perspectives. And that is really what a successful doctor-patient relationship entails—patience, trust, openness and, at times, a degree of compromise.

By interweaving my own observations as a patient and John's as a physician with those of many other doctors and patients, we feel that we have presented a balanced overview of key factors contributing to the declining trust between doctors and patients, and have identified valid, practical steps toward changing that trend.

My interviews have also uncovered some rather surprising issues contributing to frustration in the doctor-patient relationship that I believe are essential for both doctors and patients to understand. Patients need to get inside doctors' minds in order to develop realistic expectations and become empowered patients, and doctors need to get inside patients' minds in order to respond to their needs and establish productive, rewarding relationships. Each has much to gain by striving to understand the other better. If we start talking *to* each other rather than angrily *about* each other, and learn to combine good communication skills with modern technology, we'll have a powerful healing system. Both health care professionals and patients will benefit from the insights revealed by doctors and patients who were refreshingly candid about their experiences.

Some lay readers are likely to take issue with some things doctors say in these pages, and some doctors will no doubt do the same with some of the thoughts expressed by patients. But knowing what the other really thinks—and why—is a first step toward understanding.

Sound doctor-patient relationships are crucial to cutting health care costs, minimizing errors, preventing lawsuits and promoting the psychological well-being of both doctor and patient. I am pleased with the way this book has turned out and have already been rewarded for my efforts in writing it by doctors and patients who have reviewed the manuscript prior to publication and say they have gained valuable insights from reading it.

Linda Hanner

CONTENTS

1

THE UNCERTAINTY ISSUE

BOB STEPHENS TRIES to appear nonchalant as he waits nervously in the exam room for Dr. Samson to arrive. It has been over a month since his first consultation with this doctor and nearly nine months that he has been struggling with unrelenting fatigue, numbness in various parts of his body and intermittent visual disturbances. Samson, a neurologist, is the fourth physician Bob has consulted. Bob is certain the other doctors and tests have missed something, and the longer the symptoms go on the more convinced he is that his condition must be serious. He feels that if only he knew what it was, he could deal with it.

He tenses as a light tap on the door signals Dr. Samson's arrival. Samson enters smiling, sits down opposite Bob and announces, "Well, I've got good news. Your tests are normal." He seems to wait for Bob to indicate a sense of relief.

Instead, Bob's face droops and he fights to keep his voice calm. "But—there's got to be something wrong. I feel awful. I can barely function at work…"

"I really don't know what to tell you," Dr. Samson responds. "You know it's possible for depression to cause these symptoms."

"But I'm not depressed," Bob argues, his voice rising. "The tests must be missing something—are there other tests…?"

Dr. Samson interrupts in a tone betraying annoyance, "To be honest, I have already talked with the doctors you saw before me, and they weren't convinced the additional tests were necessary. I can't justify more elaborate tests at this point. I think we should consider psychological possibilities. How's the stress level in your life?"

Again, Bob denies that his symptoms could be caused by depression or stress. Dr. Samson suggests that if things don't improve he should return in a few months, leaving it up to Bob to decide if he wants to see a psychiatrist.

As Bob leaves the exam room and approaches his wife waiting in the lobby, he avoids her questioning gaze. He doesn't want to tell her it has been another wasted trip. He feels worse than he did before he came. A normally rugged man, good at coping with life's punches, he feels discouraged, helpless and angry with Dr. Samson for questioning his mental stability.

Dr. Samson is frustrated, too, knowing that Bob was upset when he left. He is really hoping he won't return. He has too many patients like Bob who seem bent on having a diagnosis and who strongly resist looking into psychological possibilities. It seems unbelievable that they apparently would rather be told they have a serious illness than talk to a psychiatrist. In medical school he was taught that close to a third of the patients who walk in his door will be suffering from psychogenic rather than physical ailments, and he is quite sure Bob is one of them—yet he knows he could be wrong.

Some diseases do take time to show up on tests. He recalls Jennifer Adams' case. Her symptoms seemed vague, too, but a repeat test six months after the initial testing revealed a brain tumor. But that doesn't happen often. Most patients like Bob go from doctor to doctor and probably never find anything medically wrong, he reassures himself.

Although in this case Bob Stephens and Dr. Samson are fictitious characters, the scenario is not uncommon, and it illustrates a key factor contributing to enormous frustration in the doctor-patient relationship. Most often, when symptoms are difficult to diagnose or treat, neither the doctor nor the patient is prepared to communicate in a manner that fosters a positive relationship. Doctors have been trained in medical school that their job is to come up with diagnoses, and patients have been conditioned to expect answers from their doctors. When that doesn't happen, blame is often assigned either to the doctor for being incompetent or to the patient for imagining or feigning symptoms.

David Hilfaker, M.D., in his book *Healing the Wounds*, poignantly describes the problems he encountered in his own practice primarily because the "fundamental issue of the uncertainty of medicine has not been addressed." He believes, and I agree, that downplaying the fallibilities of modern medicine has left both patients and physicians feeling misunderstood. After seven years of interviewing patients and medical professionals in a variety of settings, I am more convinced than ever that unrealistic expectations on the part of both are a major source of the growing antagonism between doctor and patient.

The uncertainty of medicine is a bigger reality than most

anyone is willing to admit or accept. Some estimate that three-quarters of those of us who visit a doctor have ailments that can't be immediately diagnosed or effectively treated,[1] which means that a large percentage of the patient population is in limbo at any given time. Healing of the doctor-patient relationship can't begin until patients learn to start with realistic expectations and physicians develop a better understanding of patients' psyches.

There have been a number of books written in the past ten years that have probably inadvertently reinforced the rift between doctors and patients by grossly overstating the powers of medical science. In *Bedside Manners*, historian Edward Shorter says "postmodern" medicine is characterized not only by its ability to diagnose with near certainty what's wrong with you, but to cure it as well.

To the contrary, diagnostic technology is far from perfect and the margin for human error is staggering. I don't have to go outside my own circle of family and friends to come up with a plethora of incidents in which serious medical disorders went undiagnosed or misdiagnosed for months or years. One had an adrenal gland tumor, one had a brain tumor, one had breast cancer, one had a severely deteriorating hip, one had an ovarian tumor the size of a grapefruit, one had infectious hepatitis, and the list goes on. In some instances, the problems were missed in spite of thorough examinations and extensive testing.

When such significant and obvious organic problems can go undetected by rigorously trained physicians and advanced diagnostic equipment, it isn't surprising that many more obscure and rare problems go undiagnosed for a long time. There are a number of factors that can contribute to errors and delays in making diagnoses: nonspecific symptoms, poor doctor-patient communication, lack of specific tests for some diseases, uncertain test reliability, errors in obtaining or interpreting test results or lack of physician experience in recognizing symptoms of rare diseases.

At other times, diseases present themselves in an atypical fashion causing confusion. Sharon Severson experienced symptoms of Cushing's disease for eight years before being diagnosed and appropriately treated. Although she had suffered from repeated bone fractures, bruising, cessation of menstruation (in her early thirties), weakness, protruding abdomen and other common symptoms of Cushing's disease, she had not experienced the obesity that almost invariably accompanies it. Through extraordinary will power, she had managed to keep her weight near normal. "I practically had to starve myself to keep from putting on pounds," she recalls. Because she wasn't obese, Sharon did not look like a textbook case of Cushing's disease and doctors were thrown off track.

Within the past few years I have handed out questionnaires gathering data from diagnosed patients in seven different illness groups. The results from the 232 respondents (see table next page) reinforced information gathered from thousands of interviews.

The mean (or average) length of the prediagnosis period in each group was at least two years. The MS patients had the highest average with over seven years from the onset of symptoms until the actual diagnosis. The median was also at least two years for all but one group with the lupus patients having the high median of 5.5 years, which shows at least one-half the patients in that group had gone more than five years before being diagnosed. The reasons varied. While some claimed they were not tested adequately, in most cases it just took time for the illnesses to show up on tests or for symptoms to progress to the point that physicians were able

Length of Prediagnosis Period

Data summary of Hanner survey 1993–1994

Prediagnosis period = time between onset of symptoms and correct diagnosis by a physician

A convenience sampling of 232 participants of chronic illness support groups revealed the following:

LENGTH OF PREDIAGNOSIS PERIOD

Lupus Patients
31 surveyed

Range = 2 mos.–20 years
Mean = 5.5 years
Median = 5.5 years

Lyme Disease Patients
63 surveyed

Range = 4 mos.–30 years
Mean = 2.5 years
Median = 2 years

Multiple Sclerosis Patients
23 surveyed

Range = 3 mos.–30 years
Mean = 7.05 years
Median = 2 years

Rheumatoid Arthritis Patients
26 surveyed

Range = 0–30 years
Mean = 5.05 years
Median = 2 years

Fibromyalgia Patients
60 surveyed

Range = 1 mo.–45 years
Mean = 6.8 years
Median = 2 years

Interstitial Cystitis Patients
20 surveyed

Range = 6 mos.–19 years
Mean = 7 years
Median = 3.5 years

Myasthenia Gravis Patients
9 surveyed

Range = 1 mo.–20 years
Mean = 5 years
Median = 1 year

to make a diagnosis from observable signs. (In some of these cases, physicians might have suspected a particular disease for some time, but felt it in the best interests of the patient to wait for more conclusive evidence before making the diagnosis official.)

Shorter's claim that physicians have the ability to cure most ailments is also disputable. Many illnesses such as colds and flu are self-limiting and don't require intervention. While a number of formerly deadly or treatment-resistant conditions are now curable, most chronic illnesses remain incurable and about 30 percent of the adult population in the U.S. suffers from some form of chronic illness.[2] This is due in part to advancements in medicine and sanitation which have made it possible to cure or avoid many illnesses that previously wiped out large portions of the population before they grew older and more susceptible to other less deadly yet chronic and progressive conditions such as arthritis and neurological diseases. For many chronic illnesses, deciding whether available treatments are worth the risks of long-term side effects (that might be as bad or worse than the disease) is a tough call.

In emphasizing the shortcomings of medicine, it is not my intention to put down physicians or discount the value of medical science. I have said many times that during my own experience with a long-undiagnosed illness I became acutely aware of the limitations of medical science and at the same time sincerely impressed by how much it has to offer. I would not be doing as well as I am, even writing this book, if it had not been for the work of dedicated researchers and doctors. However, the uncertainty needs to be emphasized because it has traditionally been downplayed or ignored completely. Until both health professionals and patients acknowledge and accept the reality of medicine's fallibilities, they won't be able to start learning to work together toward effective solutions.

Is Bob Stephens' illness real or imaginary? Certainly his tension is making the symptoms feel worse; tension and anxiety will aggravate virtually any medical condition. Yet, chances are good that his symptoms are not entirely a figment of his imagination, since so many illnesses do take a long time to present objective signs and be diagnosed with certainty.

I should point out that I deliberately portrayed a man in this predicament because so often it is assumed that only women feel misunderstood by their doctors. A question I am frequently asked during presentations is, "Do more women than men feel discounted by their physicians?" Although I haven't kept count, it seems that I hear from nearly as many men as women who say they were frustrated by their encounters with physicians. A male acquaintance who has a doctorate in psychology, teaches stress management and is an involved community member had many of the same complaints about the way doctors responded to him during a lengthy bout with illness as did many of the women I have interviewed.

In Bob's situation, perhaps clearcut answers won't be possible in the near future—or ever. Yet, Bob and Dr. Samson could have developed a mutually respectful relationship— one that was rewarding for Dr. Samson and therapeutic for Bob—in spite of the circumstances, if they had a better understanding of each other's needs and goals from the outset.

This book is intended to show how doctors and patients *can* work better as a team in spite of the uncertainties of medicine. It is written with the belief that a trusting, productive doctor-patient relationship can be developed regardless of whether an illness is diagnosable or curable, and regardless of whether symptoms are psychogenic or physical or a combination of both. We will look at what patients and doctors are really seeking in their relationships and how the needs of both can be met.

Chapter 2 takes a look at how American medicine has evolved since colonial times and offers some explanation for why the quality of the doctor-patient relationship has declined even though technology has advanced, and in later chapters we propose steps for improving it.

2

SET UP TO FAIL

In large part, they [American medical professionals]
achieved their goal [to become credible] by convincing soci-
ety that medicine was rooted in complex and arcane science,
that physicians, through their education, had a grasp of that
science which was unique to them as a group. It's ironic that
we are beginning to see physicians as being less than they
could be because they are too deeply rooted in science.[1]
— John M. Smith, M.D.

EVER SINCE I first published an autobiographical account of my experiences with the medical profession during my struggle with what had become a chronic illness, I have become a sounding board for people who are frustrated with doctors for one reason or another. While I was promoting my previous books, nearly every reporter and talk show host I encountered shared an off-the-air medical story about themselves, a friend or a relative. Five years later I continue to receive phone calls and letters almost daily from people with a wide array of diagnosed and undiagnosed medical problems who are unhappy with their doctors. These negative perceptions are more often based on attitudes rather than actions of physicians.

There are a number of studies that back up my own

observations. In a 1991 American Medical Association survey of public opinion, 69 percent of the respondents claimed to be losing faith in doctors,[2] and a recent Gallup Poll showed that 57 percent of those surveyed don't believe doctors care about people as much as they used to.[3] This general dissatisfaction with our society's healers is also reflected in the large number of lawsuits in which a major component is poor communication on the part of the physician.

I, too, was angry for a time about what I deemed callous and abrupt treatment from many of the physicians I encountered. However, that anger has softened as I have attempted to put myself in their shoes by researching the doctor-patient relationship from a physician's perspective and interviewing many of them personally. I have gained insights into how stressful and painful it is for doctors to try to live up to the unrealistic expectations that society has placed on them, and how difficult it is to practice medicine in an era when they must continually justify their actions to insurance companies and contend with patients who no longer trust their motives.

Clearly, patients are not the only ones who are disillusioned. Many physicians are irritated by and mistrustful of patients who they fear will sue at the slightest provocation. A disproportionate number fall victim to drug addiction, alcoholism, and suicide. According to David E. Smith, M.D., who is in charge of a California-based chemical dependency recovery center, drug abuse by doctors is four times the national average.[4] A growing number of doctors say they feel pressured, are tired of the hassles and would not choose the profession again if given a choice nor would they advise young people to do so. Minneapolis internist Gregory Silvis testifies that the scores of doctors leaving the profession is a new phenomenon: "In 1977, when I entered medical school at the University of Minnesota, I recall the dean telling us that once in medicine, nobody ever leaves."

The following revealing testimonial comes from a third-generation doctor:

> The way medicine is going today, I think it would be irresponsible to encourage a bright kid to go into it. The quality of life is terrible. You take huge responsibilities, you sink a lot of your life and money into it and it's very hard. People are angry at you. Your judgment is doubted. You have to pay a fortune in malpractice insurance. You get no feedback . . .
>
> My wife's niece is considering medical school. I think of medicine as a kind of guild, and years ago if someone's child was interested in medical school, all the other doctors would come around and help ease the way. They'd help teach and encourage that kid to get into medicine, telling them it's a great idea, a great life. But no more! Now what you hear is, "Forget it! Don't do it!" And I must admit that is what I am telling my wife's niece, and it's what I'll tell my son if he shows interest.[5]

Dr. Robert J. Wagner, a family practitioner in St. Paul, Minnesota, describes a "chronic anger" among physicians who he says often feel trapped by the pressures and responsibilities of the profession, and who are frustrated by the constraints of a system that makes it difficult to practice the way they feel is best for their patients:

> The anger encapsulates lots of things—rules and regulations . . . the physician culture. For years you put your heart and soul into training, believing you will eventually have some freedom to go out and choose your way in the world. But, it turns out not to be freedom at all. You are in service not only to your patients, but to your colleagues, the nursing staff and your own conscience. The proverbial

buck always stops with the doctor. In the worst analysis you feel trapped by the pressures and responsibilities—and the patient becomes yet another problem.

It would seem that continuing improvements in medical training and technology would be making the physician's job easier and ensuring greater satisfaction for both patients and professionals rather than increasing tension between them. Obviously, that is not the case. A glance at how the doctor-patient relationship has evolved over time amid dramatic medical advances offers some insights into why patient frustration has increased and doctors are finding the practice of medicine more difficult and less rewarding.

Colonial Medicine

Before the 20th century it was not uncommon for women to die of infections after childbirth, babies to die before reaching first birthdays and for deadly viral and bacterial illnesses to ravage entire towns. Frequent funerals for children and young adults were a harsh but accepted fact of life. Doctors of colonial times could most often offer only comforting care and make predictions concerning outcomes of conditions. No one expected any more of them.

Going back to the mid-1700s to the early 1800s, historians report that physicians were not only ineffective, they were more often than not threats to their patients. Shorter describes doctors during this period as "ruinously incompetent and aggressively meddlesome," pointing out that they were incredibly ignorant and lacking in practical experience.[6] We now see as barbaric many of the procedures that people were subjected to at the hands of doctors during earlier days of medicine—bleeding, purging with leeches, pouring hot oil on open wounds. And we shudder at the thought of going through major surgery without the aid of anesthetics as colonial patients did.

I can't help feeling bemused when Shorter, after describing in detail these early medical horrors, later puzzles over the reason that people during this era relied heavily on home remedies, calling on physicians only when death was near. He concludes that it must have been because people were more stoic and much less in tune to their bodies' physical ailments. It seems more likely that they were intelligent enough to follow their better judgment, waiting until they were sure that no remedy the doctor administered could make them feel worse than they already did. Of course they were more stoic—they didn't have any choice!

A New Era in Medicine

The 19th century brought several improvements in health care including the invention of several diagnostic tools: the stethoscope, the ophthalmoscope, the hypodermic syringe, the cystoscope and x-rays. Perhaps even more significant than the new technology was the observation in 1847 by Austrian physician Ignaz Semmelweis that death from childbed fever among young mothers in hospital wards was nearly eliminated when those who came in contact with the women washed their hands between visits. Unfortunately, Semmelweis' theory was discounted by his colleagues; women continued to die needlessly until the late 1800s when scientists discovered that microscopic organisms were the culprit in numerous diseases and could indeed be transferred from person to person. Semmelweis was right—improved hygiene made it possible to avoid transfer of infections from patient to patient. And since germs flourish in filth, overall attention to cleanliness inhibited the spread of communicable diseases such as leprosy, typhoid fever, tuberculosis, bacterial pneumonia, and bubonic plague.

The promotion of hygiene by public health officials was the main reason that life expectancy in the United States rose from almost forty to almost fifty years between 1850 and 1900. While in 1800 one-half the children had died from disease before age five, by 1900 the figure had gone down to about one-fourth.[7]

In a single century, more major medical advances had been made than had occurred in the entire previous history of civilization.[8] Throughout the latter part of the nineteenth century and into the twentieth century medical improvements continued. Scientists made the connection between vitamin deficiencies and diseases. Electron microscopes revealed that organisms much smaller than bacteria caused viral illness such as yellow fever, chicken pox, mumps, influenza, rabies, polio and the common cold. Vaccines against many of these illnesses were developed.

Miracle Medicines and Personalized Care

The use of drugs in treatment of illness evolved rapidly after World War II with the addition of an abundance of drugs to a previously modest arsenal of medicinal remedies that primarily consisted of painkillers such as morphine, aspirin, and iodine. Indisputably, the medical breakthrough of the century was the discovery of antibiotics—the so-called wonder drugs. Their development was made possible by a serendipitous discovery by Alexander Fleming. A mold blew in the window of his London lab where he was growing staphylococci bacteria, landed on his culture plate, attacked his bacteria and killed them.

Penicillin, the first of over 60 kinds of antibiotics now

available, was used to effectively treat deadly bacterial conditions: pneumonia, strep throat, scarlet fever, blood poisoning and syphilis. Antibiotics are the main reason why people in developed countries now live an average of more than twenty-five years longer than people did a century ago.

Even though many of the improvements in health care were the result of improved sanitation and chance discoveries, much of the glory was given to medical doctors who were awarded the privilege of using the new scientific technology and prescribing the miracle drugs. Equipped with tools to diagnose with greater accuracy, to perform surgery with less pain and to administer more effective medications for many conditions, physicians commanded respect, even awe, from their patients.

Along with their new-found skills and tools, for a time physicians were very accessible to their patients. Until the middle of the 20th century, they made house calls and adjusted hours to make it convenient for their patients. Dr. Fred Hafferty, professor of sociology of medicine at the University of Minnesota, Duluth, recalls seeing his physician father, who started his practice in Boston in the 1930s, only on Wednesday and Sunday nights because the rest of his father's days and evenings were devoted to patients. His physician uncle, who also started practicing during that time period, initially set up an office in his home. His patients were greeted at the door by Hafferty's aunt who chatted with them while they waited to be examined by the doctor. Those too ill to leave their beds were visited in their own homes.

The Idolization of Doctors

Perhaps even physicians at first were humbled by the rapid advances in medical technology. However, a growing sense of self-importance was almost inevitable as more rights and privileges were assigned solely to them, as medical schools became more rigid in requirements and the public continued to put physicians on a pedestal. This new breed of physician was promoted by advertisers and the media with a bombardment of promises and scare tactics that seemed designed to make society increasingly dependent on medical science. People were advised if they did not go to the doctor a serious ailment might go undetected, and if they did the doctor would find anything that was wrong in short order. A full-page magazine advertisement (duplicated in Shorter's *Bedside Manners*) sponsored by Mead Johnson and Co. in 1935 clearly illustrates how patients were conditioned. The caption reads "Only a Cold" and the ad goes on to say in part:

> And yet . . . a 'cold' may be fatal. For many a serious disease, in its early stages, masquerades as a cold . . . If all parents called the family physician immediately when a cold afflicts their children, they would be spared the grief of many a serious illness. Moreover, the few dollars spent on a visit to the physician usually brings the quickest relief from a 'common cold' and is the most economical means of caring for it.[9]

Along with dramatic improvements in sanitation and medical care came striking changes in society's attitude regarding life and death. It was no longer acceptable for people to die young. Physicians were supposed to provide answers; medical researchers were supposed to discover cures for diseases. Expectations escalated. The government invested billions of dollars in research, confident that with enough manpower and enough money medical science could fix everything. Doctors became the heroes of the day, were even revered as godlike beings. "The doctor knows best" and "Follow the doctor's orders" became popular cliches.

Millie, a woman I know who is in her seventies, provides a prime example of the patient attitude toward physicians during the earlier part of the century. She has suffered from significant health problems in recent years, some of which have mystified physicians. One day, returning from a doctor visit, she indignantly retorted, "I don't understand doctors these days. We used to be able to go see the doctor and he would know what was wrong with us right away without us having to say anything. Now we have to tell them everything and they still can't figure out what's wrong."

Being a generation or so removed from Millie and realizing this couldn't possibly be true, I tried to explain to her that physicians never did have the ability to find and fix everything, and certainly not without any input from the patient. But she remained adamant. "Yes they did! I've talked with all my friends about this and they agree. Doctors used to be smarter."

People of Millie's day were indoctrinated with the notion that doctors should and did have all the right answers. Even though physicians, in the scientific sense, are better trained now than they were fifty years ago, for people of Millie's generation that godlike image of the doctors of their youth remains fixed in their minds.

Disillusionment Sets In

Sometime between Millie's generation and the baby boomers, confidence in and respect for physicians began to wane. Medical science has continued to present new discoveries that aid diagnosis, improve surgical techniques, and make it possible to more effectively treat a variety of conditions, and patients have continued to rely heavily on physicians' skill and knowledge to resolve their medical problems. Nevertheless, satisfaction with medical care in this country has continued to decline. Looking back, five key factors stand out as components in the widening doctor-patient gap:

1—*Medical technology replaces human contact.*

First, some disillusionment surely stems from the disappointment over the loss of personal attention and time that was given to patients before medicine got on the fast track. Medical technology itself has contributed to the distancing of doctors and patients.

> Excessive use of technology has a way of desensitizing the user, especially the young, impressionable medical student, intern, resident, or new practitioner. The technology itself becomes the object of attention, of respect, of value. Test results take on a life of their own and, in composite, can become the proxy of the patient. Thus the intentions and decisions about what is and what needs to be done are between the physician (or team) and the technology.[10]
>
> —Charles B. Inlander

Others agree:

> Today there is an emotional distance, a psychological distance, perhaps even a healing distance that has been placed and left to lengthen between doctor and patient by medical technology. By using—indeed, overusing—this technology, this mechanistic wall that's been building between the care giver and the care-needy, the doctor "retreats further into his scientific cocoon," writes Louise Lander in *Defective Medicine,* and "his words and actions become less and less comprehensible to the patient, while at the same time the patient's words and actions become less and less important to the doctor's diagnosis and treatment of his condition."[11]

Medical technology has in a way replaced the doctors as the gods of medicine. People have been led to believe that there is a new magic in medical technology. This fascination with technology by patients and doctors alike often hinders the diagnostic process according to Catherine (Cate) P. McKegney, Minneapolis family practitioner:

> Much of what I have trouble with in this culture is the assumption that a test is going to provide more accurate information than my history taking. A hundred years ago Sir William Osler said that 90 percent of the time the patient will *tell* you what is wrong—and that is *still* true today. The most sensitive, most specific test I have is an accurate history. It is more sensitive than the physical exam, the CAT scan, the MRI, the blood test—or any other test ever invented.

In our fast-paced society the human quality of medicine becomes lost in the shuffling of patients from one test to another. I recall my first visit to the Mayo Clinic. The doctor in charge of my case ordered several tests. I was handed a number along with dozens of other patients lined up to wait for a chest x-ray. Our numbers were called and we were hustled along one by one to rooms to undress, don paper gowns and wait again. When our numbers were called a second time, we were shifted to new rooms and x-rayed by technicians who wasted not a second on smiles. Then we were bustled along to the next test. I was impressed with the efficiency of the system, but the process left us all feeling quite inconsequential—rather like so many head of cattle.

These days many doctors are under a great deal of pressure to see more patients in less time, to the dismay of the patients. In the earlier-mentioned survey almost 75 percent of the 232 people questioned felt their doctors did not spend adequate time with them. People of Millie's generation probably responded more favorably to their physicians partly because of the amount of time and attention they were given. During her younger days, doctors weren't so reluctant to become friends with their patients, and the caring relationship was therapeutic in itself.

A retired country doctor recalls, "Doctors used to be at a patient's beck and call. Now people must wait a week, two weeks, a month before seeing a doctor—then the visit might last a matter of minutes."

The venue of a visit with the doctor has shifted from the patient's own home to the doctor's sterile examination room. "It is not just sterile in the external sense, but also in the interactive sense," says Hafferty.

2—There has been a shift in types of illnesses.

A second element in the doctor-patient rift is that the types of illnesses that plague our society today have changed. As Hafferty points out in his book *Into the Valley: Death and Socialization of Medical Students*, we have moved beyond an era dominated by acute illnesses that your body either battled against and won or succumbed to in a relatively short period of time. As people began to live longer, the nature of the diseases predominant among people who patronized doctors' offices changed. With improved hygiene and medical intervention people are now living longer, but not without a cost, says Hafferty. "While folks just aren't dropping dead at 20, 30 and 40 years old anymore, more people are living with chronic illnesses for a good portion of their lives—40 years or more."

In fact about 30 percent of the adult population today suffers from some form of diagnosed chronic illness and

probably as many have ongoing undiagnosed conditions.[12]
Some illnesses naturally tend to develop more often later in
life, and since the population is growing older, a greater percentage will experience them. Other diseases that were often fatal 50 years ago are now managed with medication
and diet—even failing organs are replaced or kept going me-
chanically. Patients have different needs today—needs that
many physicians aren't prepared to meet. Medical school
training remains focused on dealing with acute medical problems. According to Wagner, medical schools teach a "find it
and fix it" mentality. "We are trained to make the diagnosis
and cure the problem as expediently as possible."

3—Bureaucracy threatens the doctor-patient relationship.

John Witek cites a number of other factors making the practice of medicine more difficult for physicians these days:

> Bureaucracy and the emergence of HMOs and managed
> care have added to the friction between patients and physi-
> cians. I personally believe the concept is very good, and
> critical if the United States is going to control its health
> care costs while continuing to provide quality medical ser-
> vices. The trade-off is that our actions are frequently ques-
> tioned. Physicians feel as if we are always completing forms,
> needing to explain what is being recommended. A proposed
> treatment or medication may not be approved. Then the
> patient can be frustrated and upset with the physician. The
> physician will have to explain to the patient, consider al-
> ternatives, possibly re-petition the medical insurer. This is
> time consuming and, more important, changes the tradi-
> tional patient-physician relationship into a more complex
> triad involving the insurer/health plan. Probably the num-
> ber one frustration among physicians in dealing with pa-
> tients today is that too often the encounter feels adversarial

from the onset. This altered relationship is undoubtedly a major factor. We don't feel trusted by our patients. The patient who subscribes to an HMO may come in with the preconceived notion that the physician is going to limit care because of the HMO. They may see us as advocates for the insurance company and therefore might not trust our rationale for the decisions we make. This suspicion from patients makes team work difficult.

4—*False hopes are created.*

The fourth and perhaps most significant element in the doctor-patient gap is that lay people have been set up by advertisers, media, and the medical profession to expect miracles. The transition from poorly trained, inept physicians with practically no useful diagnostic tools to well-trained physicians who are able to offer valid diagnoses and treatments happened quite rapidly. The contrast was so dramatic that medicine went through a sort of glamour period. But enough time has elapsed now for society to forget how primitive medicine used to be. A new generation of patients has evolved—one with high expectations and little understanding or acceptance of the real limitations of medicine.

We continue to hear more about the strengths of medical science than the weaknesses. Medical breakthroughs or near-breakthroughs are sensationally featured on the news even though many of them do not actually pan out. The media often gets wind of a new test or new treatment that is in the process of being developed or tested and presents it in a manner that leads the public to believe it has already been proven effective. In reality, many of these so-called breakthroughs are not able to accomplish the researchers' or inventors' goals.

For example, since Lyme disease was first identified in this country in the 1970s, there have been frequent reports by the media that a conclusive test for the disease has been developed. To date, in each case, further investigation revealed that the latest test is as fallible as the others. While writing this book I read about the availability of polymerase chain reaction (PCR) testing. It was portrayed in newspaper articles as a dramatic step forward. I contacted a University of Minnesota physician, Jesse Goodman, who has been intensely involved in research on this test and learned that it is still considered to be in the research stages. He said at this point PCR is not much more helpful than other tests in diagnosing Lyme disease since it is only relevant when used on patients who have joint inflammation, the group of Lyme patients that is already likely to test positive on other types of tests. I've also lost count of the number of acquaintances during the past six years who have commented about a media report giving the impression that a Lyme disease vaccine for humans is just around the corner. Yet each time I check directly with researchers, I'm told that it is probably still many years away.

Doctors are not living up to the promise of being able to diagnose and come up with cures for every condition. People with newly identified diseases such as AIDS can't understand why medical researchers aren't moving faster in finding more effective solutions. They are banding together and demanding that they do so.

> Today's patients expect to get well if they seek help. When they do not get well, they become angry and blame the doctor, the hospital or the government. Or they sue everyone in sight.[13]
>
> — Peter Gott, M.D.

Years ago the fallibilities and inconsistencies of medicine were not so noticeable. People generally had one family doctor who cared for them from birth. It was rare for people to be referred for second opinions. Therefore, there was no one to question or dispute a diagnosis or treatment. Since most conditions were treated by the same doctor, it was unlikely that a patient would wind up being evaluated by two, three or more physicians.

Modern transportation and increasing availability of medical specialists have made it feasible for patients to be seen by several doctors who might come up with a confusing, sometimes conflicting array of diagnoses and treatments. The patient who sees three doctors and receives three different diagnoses and treatment recommendations is beginning to learn something of the idiosyncratic nature of the diagnostic process.

> *John Witek:* Physicians are accustomed to two or more doctors having differing opinions. People who are unfamiliar with the diagnostic process tend to think ailments always fall into neat categories, obvious to a good diagnostician. This just isn't true. Often a diagnosis is not a single unchangeable entity, but rather a constantly moving target that is subject to revision in light of new information. In fact, becoming too fixated on a specific diagnosis can blind one to other valid possibilities.
>
> Even the most sophisticated medical tests will at times yield some "false positives" and "false negatives" or provide conflicting results. As in a court of law, when one is called to give a deposition, one can only say, "In my best medical opinion . . ." The diagnosis being rendered is always one's opinion based on the information currently available. In some cases clearcut answers will never be possible.

Thus, the saying "The doctor knows best" is ambiguous. It becomes a question of which doctor knows best. This was certainly true during the six years I searched for answers to the symptoms that plagued me before I was finally diagnosed and successfully treated for Lyme disease. During that time I saw over two dozen doctors, primarily specialists, who all seemed very sure of themselves, but often had conflicting opinions. Some were quite certain that my symptoms, which included involuntary movements, were psychogenic; others were convinced of the opposite. One reputable neurologist wrote in my records that "the movement appears to calm down when I'm not looking—or she thinks I am not looking." Another commented, "If this is not an organic [physical] problem, you deserve an academy award."

Even very common diseases can be confusing to doctors. As Dr. Frank Davidoff, a senior vice president of the American College of Physicians, says, "Almost no single finding in medicine points to one answer. Six doctors can look at a spot on the same chest x-ray and come up with six different opinions of what is causing it. This happens every day."[14]

A well known case of doctors having dramatically different opinions is that of pro basketball player Reggie Lewis. He was told by one group of doctors that he had a life-threatening heart condition and another that he just had a tendency to faint—to go ahead and play. His eagerness to continue playing no doubt made the latter diagnosis much more palatable. Unfortunately, Lewis' sudden death while on the basketball court appeared to prove the first doctor right, though all the facts may never be known.

Contributing to the current frustration in the doctor-patient relationship is the discrepancy in the way patients are encouraged to behave and the way that behavior is received by doctors. Among doctors I've interviewed in recent years, one of the most frequent complaints is that too many people come in with what they perceive as insignificant maladies. It seems a bit unfair that after people have been encouraged to rely on physicians for every aspect of health care, physicians have grown weary of dealing with patients who don't appear to be in dire need of medical attention.

Modern patients are really in a no-win situation in many ways. They are more educated about warning signs of diseases that can be successfully treated if caught early and are constantly advised to seek medical attention if these signs are noted. The patient whose cancer is diagnosed late is admonished for not getting regular checkups. The heart patient with advanced hardening of the arteries is told he should have sought medical attention earlier. On one hand the patient is accused of running to the doctor too frequently and on the other of not taking proper care if he or she waits too long.

5—Medical school training adds to the pain.

While patients have reason to be frustrated and perhaps angry at times, so do physicians. After all, they have been set up in a sense too—set up to fail their patients. With the emphasis in medical school on making the diagnosis, they are instilled with the notion that they should be able to find every problem and provide appropriate solutions.

> *John Witek:* The internship and residency are designed to build on one's knowledge base and diagnostic acumen, while instilling confidence in handling cases on one's own. Although an unstated purpose, some view it as a rite of passage to becoming a full-fledged physician since the training period generally becomes an endurance test—trainees are pushed close to the breaking point. No one has time to think about, let alone discuss, the best way to deliver information to the patient.

Since most internships and residencies take place in university hospitals where exotic disorders tend to be more the norm than common ailments, the physician isn't well prepared for the reality of dealing with patients in an office setting where the majority of patients come in with less dramatic, often undiagnosable problems. During my own training no one explained how to talk to patients when we couldn't provide them with an answer. Although I think that I have developed a way to deal with this issue fairly well on my own, I remember how hard it was when I first started out. If I couldn't give patients the answers they wanted I sensed their attitude to be "What kind of doctor are you?" I would try to explain that answers aren't always apparent, and that it just isn't the way you see it on television. It was difficult to deal with patients who had their own visions of what medicine is and didn't have a comprehension of its complexity.

Medical schools tend to attract people who are compulsive and perfectionistic and by nature find it difficult to admit their uncertainty or talk about their mistakes. The problem is compounded when they are not encouraged by mentors to talk about these things. The result is that many experience a great deal of inner emotional turmoil, which makes it even harder for them to establish a trusting relationship with their patients.

Dr. Cate McKegney compares the medical education system to a neglectful and abusive family system with the "grandparent" generation being represented by the chiefs of staff and senior faculty, the "parents" the attending physicians and junior faculty, and the "children" the residents and interns. In her writings she describes the medical "family" as a dysfunctional one plagued by abusive teaching methods that are being perpetuated in each new generation. She describes residency training, particularly internship, as arduous and painful—a time in which physical and emotional needs of trainees are ignored:

> They [interns] are expected, and come to expect themselves, to remain awake, stay upright, and perform responsibly for 24 to 36 hours at a time. To the rest of the world, this sounds outrageous, but the members of this family actually consider it a matter of some pride. Mood, judgment, and attentiveness are all affected. The awareness that they are becoming less competent as the night progresses contributes further to the interns' distress. Nevertheless, by the time they finish training, many have adopted the unrealistic expectations of the medical education system, unskilled at admitting human needs or human mistakes.[15]

Rather than examining which teaching methods will produce physicians who are prepared to best meet the needs of their patients, the "medical family has perpetuated the tradition of punishing training methods." Interns are required to put in 80 to 105 hours per week for a pittance. At the time of this writing I was told of one surgeon intern currently earning the equivalent of $3.50 per hour.

In an interview, Dr. McKegney discussed further the problems with the medical education system, including some of her own experiences as an intern and resident:

> Getting called by the hospital nursing staff at 3 A.M. in the midst of the half hour of sleep you're going to get that night to be asked to give an order for medication to help a patient sleep—that's the quintessential affront. I remember standing over many a person's hospital bed and thinking, You know, if you moved over a just a little, tiny bit, I would lie down and sleep on your bed—you don't even have to get out of the bed. All I wanted to do with every cell in my body was sleep. Nothing else. Just sleep. All things during residency came down to the question: Is it worth losing an

hour of sleep to do this? Some people spend five to seven years in residency. That's a lot of time to spend thinking about whether or not you're going to get enough sleep.

If you ask physicians in training to learn to be attentive to their patients' psychological needs, but ignore their own physical or psychological needs, you have a losing proposition. There is no way on God's green earth that somebody who eats bad food, doesn't sleep enough and doesn't get to sleep with his or her spouse is going to be able to care about somebody else's psychological needs. Yet, that is what we are asking medical trainees to learn to do; we are demanding that they be superhuman in ways that we have not previously demanded, which is really cruel.

In addition to the physical pain inflicted by strenuous schedules, interns are subjected to a system in which clear feedback is rare and "correction is more common than affirmation," leaving the medical trainee feeling incompetent, said McKegney, adding:

> Receiving punishing comments about mistakes teaches trainees to hide errors, by lying if necessary . . . The medical trainee system functions like a rigid family when trainees are given responsibilities beyond their abilities or are not allowed to increase their independence when developmentally ready. The system rigidly assigns duties to house staff by year of training, disregarding previous experience or individual talents. In their first month, interns are traditionally given the same responsibilities as those carried by their immediate predecessors with 12 months of experience—an unrealistic expectation.[16]

Dr. McKegney suggests that physicians need to heal their own wounds from their training before they can "parent" differently within the medical training system, and teach other physicians to better respond to patients' emotional needs.

Hope for the Future

Having already gone through some significant changes, the doctor-patient relationship in this country is again in a state of transition. How we all deal with the contributing issues will determine whether the current sense of frustration will worsen or improve.

Some professionals argue that it is impossible to give patients the time and attention that early physicians did—that physicians shouldn't be expected to also be counselors, and they can't worry about every patient's emotional needs. As one doctor put it, "The doctor's training and responsibility are primarily for the patients' physical well-being, not for helping them emotionally and mentally."

I would respond that although actual counseling does take time, not much more time needs to be spent with each patient to help him or her deal with the emotional and psychological components of illness. Simple things, like choice of wording, often make a big difference. By improving care—even perceptions of care—through better communication and increased understanding on the part of both physicians and patients, satisfaction for both can be significantly increased. When satisfaction increases, less time and money will be spent on legal battles, and the saved money and time can be used to further improve the quality of care.

While I understand that physicians don't have the time or expertise to act as psychotherapists, it will be helpful for them to understand how manner and choice of wording can significantly impact a patient's sense of well-being. The cost of not addressing emotional and psychological issues is high. When patients are unhappy with care, they are less likely to follow through on or respond well to suggested treatments, they are more likely to engage in doctor-shopping (which is likely to increase the probability of unnecessary repeat tests) and they are more likely to consider lawsuits.

As the rift between doctors and patients grows, we must consider what can be done to change the trend. By exploring what both physicians and patients really want and need, a plan for working together toward healing the doctor-patient relationship will become clearer.

3

What Patients Want Most from Doctors

I attribute my successful management of this illness and im-
measurably improved quality of life to finding a physician
who consistently respected and believed what I had to say . . .
By working with me, rather than in spite of me, he was able
to diagnose and begin to treat my disease.[1]

—Eileen Radzuinas

WHETHER PEOPLE respond to their doctors with a sense of admiration or indignation will depend on more than competency and bedside manner. Of course everyone would like to have a physician who is technically skilled as well as compassionate and understanding. Yet what people want most depends a great deal on circumstances. After many years of listening to people discuss their medical woes and describe their doctor experiences, I have recognized that those who visit doctors for symptom evaluation or treatment can generally be categorized into one of four groups: repair seekers, reassurance seekers, diagnosis seekers, or health management seekers. One might find oneself in different categories at different times.

The Repair Seekers

Several summers ago, while mowing the lawn, I mindlessly reached down to pull out a lump of grass lodged in the chute of the running mower. As soon as I felt the thud of the blade hitting my thumb, I realized my folly and a quick glance at the results convinced me that a doctor could be useful. Since I immediately passed out, I was fortunate that my husband was home to phone our family doctor, who, even though it was a weekend, agreed to meet us at his clinic a few miles away. Within a short time he had the deep, gaping wound stitched, and I was on the road to recovery. Later I developed an infection in the wound which the doctor promptly treated with antibiotics. Although the injury was relatively minor, the incident raised the doctor to hero status in my mind.

Likewise, I was appreciative when after more than 12 hours of unproductive labor with my fourth child, who was determined to enter the world breech, that the doctor in charge had the knowledge and skill required to perform a caesarean section. He had to work quickly since my blood pressure dropped dangerously low once the anesthetic was administered. He delivered our healthy eight-pound, six-ounce son, and I recovered from the surgery without complications, reinforcing my appreciation of modern medical technology and competent physicians.

These two incidents define the type of situations for which the first group of patients, the repair seekers, request help. Individuals in this group might have lacerations, broken bones, acute infections or other medical conditions that a physician is likely to quickly and accurately assess and go about repairing. The wounds are stitched, the bones are set or appropriate medications are administered.

Surely, these are the kinds of conditions that are most likely to draw respect and appreciation from patients while providing satisfaction for physicians as well. In his book *Health and Healing: Understanding Conventional and Alternative Medicine,* Andrew Weil, M.D., points out that traditional medicine is at its best when treating acute illnesses and handling medical emergencies. It is these predicaments which medical school has done a good job teaching doctors to handle.

Although ideally the repair seekers would find a doctor who is both proficient and sympathetic, competency is most likely at the top of the list. As long as the physician responds to the immediate needs and does so properly, one is not likely to gripe about a doctor's poor bedside manner.

The Reassurance Seekers

The second group, the reassurance seekers, on the other hand, consult the doctor for symptoms that generally are not life-disrupting and need less immediate attention. They include those who have a nagging symptom, perhaps stomach discomfort, chronic headaches, back pain—symptoms that are not usually severe enough to disrupt their lives significantly, but are persistent enough to eventually prompt them to consult a doctor.

For instance, Paul, who is in his mid-forties, had been experiencing a racing heartbeat and chest discomfort off and on for some time. Knowing that his father had died of a heart attack in his early 50s, he finally decided to make an appointment with an internist to see if anything serious might be brewing. When a thorough physical exam, including an EKG and stress test, showed his heart to be in good working order, he became less concerned about the symptoms. Since he normally drank several cups of coffee a day, his doctor also suggested that he cut back on caffeine, which indeed seemed to resolve his symptoms. Once Paul was reassured that nothing serious was wrong he stopped worrying about his symptoms.

Jane is another example of a reassurance seeker. She wondered if she might have an ulcer because of frequent stomach distress. She looked up causes of similar symptoms in her family medical book which described some potentially serious causes, even cancer. A thorough examination and some tests showed that esophagitis (inflammation of the esophagus) was most likely the cause of her symptoms. Her doctor instructed her to sleep with her upper body slightly elevated and take antacids. These measures helped. Once she knew the cause, even though she didn't always take proper care to avoid flare-ups, she was able to put up with them knowing the problem wasn't life-threatening.

Providing they are convinced their doctors have done a thorough exam and offered reasonable explanations, reassurance seekers are likely to be satisfied with their doctor encounters as well. Again, competency is their main concern. Once they have been reassured by a doctor they perceive as trustworthy, they are likely to go on with their lives and either learn to avoid activities that aggravate their aches and pains or live with them.

The Diagnosis Seekers

The third patient category, the diagnosis seekers, includes those who have ongoing symptoms that are disrupting their lives to a greater degree. Perhaps pain is keeping them awake at night to the point they are no longer functioning well during the day. They might be missing work or have been forced to cut back on other activities they accomplished easily before their symptoms started. Often they have visited several doctors who have not been able to provide answers. Yet the symptoms continue to disrupt their lives.

Recalling the data from the survey discussed in Chapter 1 which showed the prediagnosis period is frequently a matter of months or years, it seems likely that a significant segment of the patient population is in such a predicament at any given time.

Diagnosis seekers are looking not only for a competent physician, but one that will validate their symptoms, then reassure them that they won't be abandoned before a diagnosis is found. Kindness, compassion, and patience become central to building a trusting relationship between doctor and patient.

Health Management Seekers

The fourth category of patients, health management seekers, are those who were at one time diagnosis seekers, but now have a confirmed chronic illness. Unlike the repair seekers, their symptoms cannot easily be fixed through surgical procedures or medication. Finding the best protocol for managing symptoms might involve a long process of trial and error and as their conditions worsen (or improve) their needs will change. Qualities such as patience and compassion will be important to them.

In the absence of gross negligence or incompetence which would alarm any patient, the diagnosis seekers and the health management seekers are least likely to be satisfied with their physician encounters. And of those two groups, the diagnosis seekers, the Bob Stephenses described in the first chapter of this book, are the ones whose needs are least likely to be met. These are the cases that provide the biggest challenge for physicians and are most likely to call for perseverance. Several doctors I interviewed admitted that people who have complicated symptoms are intimidating. St. Paul internist John C. Butler says:

> The typical competitive, success-oriented physician finds it unpleasant to admit that he is not going to be able to resolve a problem. It becomes easier to assign blame to the patient. In my own mind, I still struggle to look upon these patients as a challenge and not a source of frustration. I tell myself that I will have achieved success if I have been able to make them feel better, even if I can't diagnose the problem. We have to learn to distinguish looking for a disease from treating the illness. It is easy to forget how the illness is affecting the patient.

Depending on the type of patient, the physician can fill several roles including that of healer, encourager, health manager or medical detective. No matter what the role, the physician can have a powerful therapeutic effect that will impact the patient's recovery or ability to manage symptoms as well as his or her overall sense of well-being. A patient can walk out of a doctor's office feeling devastated or uplifted based simply on the doctor's manner or choice of wording.

More than anything, I hope this book will help physicians see how they can help their patients whether or not they are able to provide a specific diagnosis or treatment, and patients to see how they can facilitate more productive and rewarding relationships with their doctors.

Upcoming chapters provide many more specific examples of doctor-patient interactions, contrasting those that were helpful with those that were not.

4

STARTING OFF ON
THE RIGHT FOOT

*To be ill is a trial under any circumstances, but to be ill and not
know the cause is a particularly great affliction. The burden
imposed by such a situation is not merely being without access to a cure. There's the added fear of the unknown, isola-
tion from not knowing other people who have gone through
the same thing and, worst, self-blame, aided by the medical
profession's failure to understand what you're experiencing.* [1]
—Jenifer A. Nields, M.D.

NATIONALLY THERE has been increasing interest and attention given to psychosocial skills among
physicians. For the past 12 years an organization
called the American Academy on Physician and Patient,
which consists of physicians and other medical professionals from around the country, has been sponsoring courses to
train physicians who teach at medical schools so they in turn
can teach students how to establish a good rapport with their
patients. (See Appendix for more about this organization.)

Some medical schools are adopting educational programs
designed to teach compassion and empathy. Residents and
medical students at Hunterdon Medical Center in
Hunterdon, New Jersey, take part in a course during which
they are assigned false identities and for a day play the role
of patients with various infirmities. With the goal of becoming

more in tune to patients' needs, they are subjected to interviews and examinations to simulate the experience of actual patients.[2]

These endeavors are important and medical students testify they are gaining insights which they believe will ultimately help them become more caring physicians. However, at this point these training programs are focused on the post-diagnosis period—the time after the patient has already been diagnosed with a serious condition such as cancer, arthritis or AIDS. By ignoring the prediagnosis period, the time between the onset of symptoms and the actual diagnosis, medical professionals are missing a crucial opportunity to establish trust at the outset, and to set a pattern that will encourage open communication throughout the course of the illness. Instead, reservations and misunderstandings during the prediagnosis period often set the stage for continuing deterioration of communication. Once this happens it is difficult to redirect interactions to a more positive mode.

As discussed in the first chapter, for some types of disorders the time before the diagnosis is often prolonged (lasting several years), but even when it is relatively short (a matter of months) many patients confide that it is the most traumatic time of the illness for themselves and their families. The needs of the patient during this time have generally not been recognized or addressed by the medical profession. There has been a tendency to deny the reality of the symptoms and the associated psychological stress until a concrete physical diagnosis can be established.

Paul J. Donoghue, Ph.D., and Mary E. Siegel, Ph.D., in their book *Sick and Tired of Feeling Sick and Tired: Living with Invisible Chronic Illness*, make the assertion that "the degree of mental anguish that an individual will suffer from his illness, as well as the amount of care, trust, respect and compassion he will receive, is dependent on three factors outside himself."³

One of the three factors they list is clarity of the diagnosis. In other words, if an illness doesn't have a name, people tend to question the reality of it and are sometimes unwilling to make allowances for that person's inability to carry on normally. (The other factors listed are social acceptability of the disease and potential severity of the symptoms.)

Of the earlier-mentioned 232 patients surveyed, over 60 percent of them said they were treated with more compassion by doctors after their illness was validated by a diagnosis. Among the six different illness groups studied, the lupus group had the highest percentage of people who felt this way at 83 percent. The following graph shows the remaining percentages:

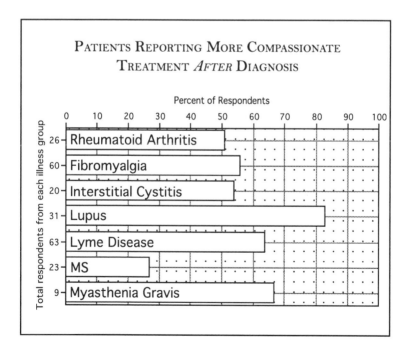

PATIENTS REPORTING MORE COMPASSIONATE
TREATMENT *AFTER* DIAGNOSIS

The way a physician responds to the patient during the prediagnosis period can significantly impact how well the patient manages symptoms. This is illustrated by the following story which was shared in a letter from Harold (not his real name), a Wisconsin man:

> On November 20, 1990, I became dizzy, very weak and began having tremors. I finished up at work and had difficulty driving home. By morning, walking had become difficult and slow. It was no longer automatic; it seemed to require thought. I would invariably angle off to the right, or fall to the right or backwards. The tremors were still present, my entire body jerked randomly, and I experienced terrible nystagmus [rapid involuntary movement] in my eyes.
>
> That afternoon my family doctor examined me and declared I had an inner ear infection. He prescribed antibiotics and Antivert, neither of which gave me any relief. A few days later he decided to try Scopolamine, but it did not help either.
>
> I was referred to an ENT specialist who ordered a comprehensive audiologic exam and blood work. Nothing out of the ordinary showed up.
>
> In mid-December my family doctor ordered a CT scan of my head. Everything was normal. Based on this and on negative results from further blood work he still suspected an inner ear infection. By this time I was much less sharp mentally. I had to think about simple things like correct spelling for the first time in my life, and I had trouble remembering phone numbers and addresses.
>
> I was sent to a neurologist who ordered more blood work and an MRI of my head. Again, everything was negative or normal. He suspected either MS, or an emotional basis for the symptoms, and put me on Klonopin, which only made me incontinent.

In January I returned to the neurologist for a followup exam. He had decided, based on my December appointment and the results of the tests, that my symptoms were the result of an "obsessive, maladaptive personality" and "stress." He criticized everything about my life. He asked why I was living at home with my parents at age 35 and why I had such a low-paying job and suggested that everything about my life was stressing me. He went so far as to state that my chorea was "intentional." He put me on Xanax and recommended counseling.

I did not believe the stress theory for an instant, since I have a strong personal faith, and I am basically satisfied with my life. I felt angry and betrayed. I took the Xanax for a time, but I gradually eased myself off around the end of March because I knew it was habit-forming and because I could not see that it was helping my symptoms.

At about that time I went for a psychological assessment in order to be put on social security disability and to receive Medicaid. A week later the psychologist's report arrived stating that my symptoms were the result of a "conversion disorder": I was consciously or subconsciously manufacturing the symptoms in order "to get attention or to avoid responsibility." It also stated that his diagnosis was based on his 30-minute assessment and on the conclusions of the previous neurologist.

In September 1991 I finally saw a physician at the Mayo Clinic who was both a neurologist and a psychiatrist. After a thorough neurological exam and interview she diagnosed my condition as "vestibular neuronitis with aggravation by medication." In other words, I had either a bacterial or viral infection of the eighth cranial nerve, which serves the inner ear. And I was told that the most effective treatment was time. All I needed was time to get better! No counseling was needed, no tranquilizer would help. The problem could recur at any time, or might never occur again. According to her, the Xanax had held back my recovery and the doctors had been "way off the mark" in prescribing it and in recommending counseling for what was obviously a physical problem.

My recovery has continued since then to the point where on January 20, 1992, I was able to return to work. I have done well, but must watch that I do not become too tired. If I push myself too hard, the symptoms tend to return.

In Harold's case the physicians had done their part. They had ordered what they felt were pertinent tests and had tried several medications. When tests failed to reveal answers and medications didn't help, it was decided that the problem was psychogenic. Harold did what anyone who is suffering from symptoms serious enough to put him out of commission would do—convinced that his symptoms had a physical basis, he continued to seek help.

Ironically, the initial diagnosis by Harold's family doctor was probably accurate, since vestibular neuronitis translates to an inner ear infection in lay language. The problem was not in the doctor's diagnostic acumen, but in his failure to gain Harold's trust in the diagnosis, and to reassure him that the problem would probably improve with time. Not only did the medication he prescribed fail to help, it may have been the culprit of what Harold perceived to be a worsening of his condition (loss of mental sharpness, memory problems, etc.), which in turn became a source of alarm for him. One can only speculate, but if the doctor(s) had handled his case more tactfully early on, it might have been less complicated and costly and less traumatic for Harold.

Even though the Mayo doctor who diagnosed his condition was not able to provide medication to correct his problem, the diagnosis was a turning point. By acknowledging the reality of his symptoms, the physician gained Harold's trust and he was able to take his focus off proving he was sick. Assured that nothing else could be done medically, he was able to concentrate on managing his condition. He recuperated sufficiently to return to work. Prior to the diagnosis, his frustration with physicians and anxiety about whether or not he would be abandoned by them had caused more stress and, since stress aggravates any medical condition, he probably felt worse physically.

The physician was not able to play the role of healer in Harold's case, but she was able to play the roles of detective and encourager. In the eyes of some physicians, her diagnosis was still somewhat nebulous since it could not be confirmed by a medical test. But the fact that she validated Harold's symptoms and was able to offer an explanation that was plausible to him enabled him to start living a more productive life in spite of his health problems.

Patients who have been diagnosed with chronic illness often say that the time between the onset of symptoms and the diagnosis was the worst, even when the disease is serious and the prognosis is poor. When patients are encouraged to deny the reality of their symptoms it becomes very difficult for them to move on to a point of acceptance. I eventually came to terms with my situation before I was diagnosed, but it took me nearly five years to do so. Had I understood the diagnostic process better, much frustration might have been avoided.

Establishing Mutual Trust During the Prediagnosis Period

From their first meeting, both patient and doctor have responsibilities in establishing the tone and quality of their relationship.

THE DOCTOR'S ROLE

By briefly recounting some events from my own experience, perhaps I can give a clearer picture of the way physicians can either help or hinder a patient's ability to successfully manage symptoms before the diagnosis.

Very early in my illness I was told by my family physician that I had "too many symptoms" to be believable, which from the outset put me on guard about what to tell other doctors about my symptoms. Within the first month, I was referred to a neurologist who put me through a series of tests. I waited two months for the results, only to learn they had not offered a clue as to the cause of my condition which included numb sensations, generalized body pain, urinary frequency, extreme weakness and uncoordinated gait.

After explaining the test results, the neurologist admitted that he was quite certain my problems were due to neurosis since nothing had shown up on the tests, and an MMPI had shown me to have a hysterical personality. (Shortly afterward I was evaluated in person by a psychologist; tests she gave me came back within the normal range. Also, a few years later an MMPI at the Mayo Clinic showed me to have a stable personality.) The neurologist did offer that there was a "slight" chance he could be wrong and went on to say, "I could refer you to another neurologist for another opinion, but someone else's tests won't be any better and they aren't likely to find anything more—anyway, most people who go from doctor to doctor looking for answers are hypochondriacs."

Those comments were the first of many made by doctors that undermined my self-confidence and added to my anxiety about consulting new physicians.

(Incidentally, Dr. Grant Dahlstrom, head of the Department of Psychology at the University of North Carolina and coauthor of two handbooks on the use of the Minnesota Multiphasic Personality Inventory, states that the MMPI should be used with extreme caution in situations concerning undiagnosed physical conditions and only in conjunction with other psychological tests.)

Although I understand that psychogenic possibilities need to be considered, the neurologist's approach was not the best even if my symptoms had been the result of a neurosis. My life had been thrown into an uproar, my body was screaming that something was terribly amiss, and the doctor that I had accepted as an authority on illness was telling me there was no point in looking any further for a physical cause. As in Bob Stephens' case, my doctor was expecting me to be pleased that nothing serious was showing up on tests, but to me that just meant the tests were missing something.

The anxiety and apprehension I felt around doctors no doubt contributed to the perceptions of many of them that I was neurotic. I became uncertain of how much to tell and how much not to tell so as not to have my symptoms discounted entirely. Every time I entered a doctor's office I feared I would be viewed as mentally unbalanced based on the first doctor's opinion about me. I became more focused on my symptoms even as I questioned my ability to assess them. That continuous self-doubt and fear was emotionally draining and the accompanying tension made my physical symptoms more intense and harder to manage.

My experience might have been less stressful had the initial doctor responded differently. The illness probably still would have taken a long time to diagnose since at the time little was known about Lyme disease, but those years might have been less traumatic.

Almost four years into my illness I was introduced to Dr. John Witek, who worked with me on managing symptoms while we continued to search for answers during the last few years I was ill. It was through the relationship that we developed that I realized it is possible for doctors and patients to work as a team. It was a new experience for me to have a doctor who consistently encouraged my input and involvement in the decision making regarding my care. While I had previously been apprehensive about visits to doctors, I looked forward to my appointments with him knowing that I would most likely leave with a boosted ego and feeling more relaxed about my symptoms, rather than feeling defeated and discouraged. In the tangible sense, he didn't really do any more for me than many of the other doctors. He prescribed medications in attempts to alleviate symptoms, but so had many others. He referred me to other specialists from time to time, but so had some others. He was not even the doctor who made the diagnosis or successfully treated me. However, he conveyed a sincere desire to do his best to help me, and although he was not the doctor who diagnosed or treated me, I consider him instrumental in the process. He gave me the courage not to give up and helped me to accept my situation before the diagnosis.

I don't want to leave the impression that the dozens of doctors I encountered earlier in my illness were bad doctors. In fact, most of them were well trained and conscientious. It was subtle things like choice of wording and manner that made a very big difference. Based on my experiences and those of other patients who have developed a positive rapport with their doctors, I offer the following suggestions for physicians during the prediagnosis period:

Empathize with the patient.

On our first encounter, following the history-taking and

exam, John commented, "This must be terribly frustrating for you. You deserve some answers. I hope we'll be able to help you." To this day, eight years later, I get emotional when I think how grateful I was to hear those words. It was the first time in nearly four years of dealing with an unnamed illness that anyone in the medical profession had verbally empathized with my predicament. The positive impact of those few sentences on my emotional state was enormous.

It seems that many doctors are afraid of feeding into what they think might be a neurotic desire for attention by offering empathy in the face of uncertainty. Doctors who are careful not to establish a physical diagnosis until they are very sure are sometimes relatively nonchalant when it comes to psychological labeling. This often creates more emotional anguish than they will ever know. Although psychological factors need to be considered, a great deal of tact is in order. Chapter 7 discusses how to handle uncertain situations and how to help patients understand the need to look at psychogenic possibilities.

Validate the patient's symptoms.

Whether symptoms are more physical or psychological in nature and whether or not any abnormalities show up on tests, the symptoms and concerns are real to the patient who is experiencing them.

Author and speaker Sefra Pitzele was ill for several years before being diagnosed with systemic lupus erythematosus. She describes going to several doctors who responded to her abruptly until finally finding a physician she trusted to work with her until she found a diagnosis. On the first visit, following the examination, that physician announced, "Sefra, I don't know whether your symptoms are physical, psychological or a combination of both. But you and I are going to stick together until we get to the bottom of this."

This doctor accomplished several important objectives in just a few sentences. He validated her symptoms without closing the door on any possible causes. He clinched her trust in him by confirming that she would be involved in the process. Knowing that he wasn't jumping to hasty conclusions concerning either her mental state or her physical condition and that her own ideas and feelings would not be discounted, she felt confident in working with him. When he promised to continue working with her "until we get to the bottom of this," she felt reassured that he would not give up out of boredom or frustration.

Reassure that the patient won't be abandoned.

I suspect that many patients who are searching for a diagnosis are also seeking, even more than the diagnosis, reassurance that they won't be abandoned. They fear no one will help them until they have a diagnosis.

> After many years, I have come to realize it hasn't been the diagnosis that I've been seeking. I only wanted to be believed and offered some sort of help for my symptoms. I mistakenly believed that my disease needed a name before help would be offered.
> —Kathy Birdwell, Chandler, Arizona

When I felt reassured that John was willing to stick with me and help me to manage symptoms, having a name for my illness became less important. I never left the office that he didn't invite me to call if anything came up between visits. Knowing that I had his verbal permission to do so was incredibly reassuring. While some physicians might fear a barrage of calls if they encourage patients to do so, I believe the opposite often occurs. When I had been seeing doctors who did not encourage phone calls, each time my symptoms worsened I would fret about whether the doctor would be annoyed or think I was foolish if I called. My anxiety would spiral as I thought, What if this keeps getting worse and the doctor doesn't believe me? I would become tense and feel worse and on occasion I would call, probably sounding like a basket case when I did because I was so nervous. When I knew it was okay to call if necessary, I was more relaxed when the symptoms intensified or a new symptom appeared. The symptoms almost invariably settled down again, and rather than making the call, I made notes about the occurrence to discuss on the next visit. Even though the visits were usually scheduled several months apart, it was reassuring to know that my situation would be reevaluated periodically by a caring doctor, and I would have the opportunity to air my concerns.

Acknowledge limitations.

> I am convinced medicine would take a giant step forward if its practitioners could let down their hubris and help patients develop reasonable and realistic expectations about doctors' skills. Self-honesty could go a long way toward resolving the incompatibility between real doctors in a real world and professional actors in imaginary stories.[+]
>
> —Peter Gott, M.D.

Recently, I was asked to join a committee to plan a series of workshops for a women's retreat. During one of our meetings I brought up the possibility of including one on patients' rights and responsibilities which would, in part, discuss the many reasons illnesses often take a long time to diagnose. One woman's immediate response was, "Well, the reason it takes a long time to diagnose so many illnesses is that doctors are incompetent!" Her comment was followed by nods in agreement.

As I attempted to explain that illnesses take a long time to diagnose for many reasons and that most often the length of the prediagnosis period has nothing to do with the doctor's competency, I realized that the attitudes of these women were based on misunderstandings which have been fostered by the lack of openness and honesty from physicians about the limitations of medical science. That was one of the things that bothered me most about my experience with a long undiagnosed illness—so many of the physicians spoke with so much certainty about things that were so uncertain. I was given the impression that if nothing showed up on tests, there couldn't be anything wrong. Until I met John no one had taken time to explain that some diseases have no specific tests, that many diseases take a long time to diagnose and that sometimes a diagnosis can be made only after observing a situation over a long time. He admitted that even the most sophisticated medical tests can yield false results, either positive or negative. Had a doctor taken time to explain these things earlier in the illness it would have been helpful to me and my family.

Most people find openness and honesty admirable qualities in a physician. Laurence A. Savett, a 30-year veteran of the practice of primary care internal medicine in St. Paul, verifies that sharing uncertainty "validates and enriches the partnership between doctor and patients," adding that "most people can handle the truth very well."

In order to develop realistic expectations, patients need to understand the complexities of the diagnostic process— that some conditions might never be diagnosable. They also need to know that finding the best treatment might involve a long process of trial and error.

John Witek: Often patients don't realize how complex and uncertain the diagnostic process can be in certain instances. It's essential for them to have an understanding of this so they might be better prepared to accept the reality of what doctors can and can't do.

Be honest, yet sensitive.

Physicians might at times suspect a specific disease, but may not want to risk upsetting a patient by mentioning it until there is more certainty. Although honesty is important, discerning how much to tell can be difficult.

John Witek: I think it is important to be up front with patients. When answers aren't clear, I explain from the outset that I am not likely to quickly resolve the issue for them. I don't intend to give an answer when I am not sure of a diagnosis and I refuse to make one up. For instance, I might see a patient who has had one MS-like episode and a brain-imaging study shows a lesion or lesions typical for this diagnosis. This would not meet the criteria for a diagnosis of MS, and I wouldn't want to alarm the patient at that point. Just mentioning the possibility of MS can cause anxiety in many because of perceptions of this disease by the general population. These cases need to be handled discreetly; I surely don't have all the answers about the best way to approach patients. It is difficult to balance issues such as honesty with the patient versus the potential emotional impact of some of the words and diagnoses we mention, especially if not yet well-defined.

Encourage patient involvement.

While some patients might want their physician to make all the decisions for them, the attitude of most patients today is to want to be informed and involved in their care.

John Witek: If the initial evaluation and tests don't lead to a specific diagnosis, I tell the patient it isn't unusual not to come up with many answers on the first few visits. I might then offer some options. We can either watch the symptoms over a period, consider further tests, try some medications or refer the patient to another physician for a second opinion. How far the issue is pursued often depends on how the patient feels about it. I might tell the patient, "I am not in your body and am not experiencing the symptoms. You have to tell me if there is something that needs to be done now or not." This helps empower the patient and might make him or her feel more a part of the process. Often people will choose to simply monitor symptoms for a period when they know they aren't going to be abandoned.

Dr. Wagner has found that encouraging patients to play an active role is helpful. He accomplishes this by assigning "homework" tasks for them to do between visits:

If they say they are waking up at night all sweaty, I tell them to take their temperature and record it when they wake up. If they feel they are losing weight, I tell them to weigh themselves at specific times every day. That way, the next time they come in, rather than a lot of vague complaints, they have more well-defined symptoms for me to evaluate.

Keep an open mind.

It is important for doctors to keep an open mind when evaluating patients, rather than putting too much store in opinions of previous doctors. I often hear from patients who were finally diagnosed simply because they had found a physician who evaluated them independently of others' conclusions. Doctors who do so stand a better chance of thinking of possibilities that others have missed.

As an example, a friend of mine went through extensive

testing for debilitating weakness and fatigue. Although none of the tests showed anything blatantly abnormal, her family physician noted that her aldosterone levels were at the high end of the normal range. He referred her to an endocrinologist who further evaluated her symptoms and test results, decided they were insignificant and diagnosed her symptoms as stress-induced. I suspect that many doctors would have taken the specialist's diagnosis as the final word. Fortunately, this woman's doctor didn't. Six months later he ordered a repeat CAT scan, which revealed an adrenal gland tumor. It was surgically removed and the woman recovered nicely.

Avoid blaming the patient.

There are times when it is fairly obvious that a patient's actions are contributing to his illness and he perhaps needs to be made aware of this in a tactful way. Such might be the case in people who smoke or drink heavily, or do not take proper care with serious medical conditions like diabetes or heart conditions. However, in many cases patients are blamed for bringing on their conditions when they have little or no control over what is happening to their bodies. Rather than empowering the patient to get better, blaming compounds anguish in an already difficult situation.

> I was ready to forgive him [the doctor] for not being able to find out what was wrong with me. But I didn't expect him to turn on me and accuse me of being the one to cause my own problems. When he did, I felt incredibly betrayed.
> —nurse/lupus patient

THE PATIENT'S ROLE

Although I am convinced the advice outlined in this chapter will be helpful to doctors in establishing trust during the prediagnosis period, I am also aware that it is important for patients to do their part to help the doctor help them. When my own attitude changed, when I became less defensive and more confident in myself, I noticed a big difference in the way doctors responded to me. They, in turn, seemed more relaxed and to even enjoy working with me as a patient.

When I speak to patients about the prediagnosis period I offer the following suggestions:

Be assertive, but not demanding.

While it is important for patients to be assertive when it comes to getting their questions answered about medical tests and treatments and letting their doctors know they want to be involved in decision making, there is a difference between being assertive and demanding more than is humanly possible.

It is not easy for a patient to be in limbo, but inability to provide a diagnosis can be disconcerting for physicians as well. Establishing trust and effective rapport before the diagnosis takes a certain amount of tolerance and understanding from both physician and patient. Those who insist on definitive answers when tests are inconclusive or who become hostile when a physician doesn't say what they want to hear only make a difficult situation worse.

I spoke with one woman who admitted to slapping her physician across the face. Another man became so frustrated with his physician that he started yelling at him, was escorted out of the office and told not to come back. These patients run the risk of alienating the entire medical profession; as word gets around, no doctor will want to deal with them.

Patients deserve explanations when doctors don't agree with their ideas or suggestions, but it is not fair for them to pressure doctors into prescribing a test or treatment, or to provide a diagnosis that he or she does not believe is appropriate.

Strive for acceptance.

Often, those with undiagnosed illness become focused on proving they are sick, which might not even be possible, rather than finding the best possible solutions under the circumstances. It is understandable that people want a diagnosis quickly. But when it is apparent that the prediagnosis period could extend to months or years, they need to try to refocus. That doesn't mean giving up on having an answer or on pursuing possibilities as they come to light; it just means learning to take things a day at a time and living as full and productive a life as possible in the meantime. It took me over four years before I was finally able to reach a point of acceptance with my undiagnosed illness, but once I did I experienced a tremendous joy and sense of inner peace in spite of the uncertainty and debilitating symptoms that continued for another two years before I was diagnosed.

Don't blame doctors for what is beyond their control.

Again, the notion that someone should be blamed when a diagnosis can't be made needs to be set straight if the animosity between physicians and patients is ever to be resolved. I lost count of the times that people exclaimed, "You mean they still haven't figured out what's wrong with you?"— implying there must be something wrong with the doctors I was seeing or with me. Although doctors can be incompetent, and patients can be uncooperative, too often blame is assigned to either the doctor or patient when it shouldn't be. Not everything shows up on tests. Many diseases have no specific tests, and it might take a long period of observation before a diagnosis can be made. A friend's mother doctored for nearly eight years before Parkinson's disease could be conclusively diagnosed.

Some doctors are particularly good at working with difficult-to-diagnose patients. In fact, John says he finds these cases "can at times be intellectually stimulating and challenging." However, my conversations with doctors suggest that a more typical personality of those who choose medicine, combined with the extensive scientifically oriented training, makes for doctors who would generally rather deal with something quantifiable.

It is clear that both patients and physicians need to be open-minded during the prediagnosis period, and there must be a willingness to discuss possibilities and perhaps make some compromises. It is refreshing to hear stories from doctors and patients who have resolved differences once they have been aired and have developed positive relationships even before the diagnosis. It can be done!

5

PATIENTS' TOP 10 COMPLAINTS ABOUT DOCTORS

B ECAUSE MEDICINE is not an exact science, because people's bodies are unique and because doctors are human, it will never be possible for doctors to consistently make medical decisions that are in the best interests of their patients, or to perform every medical procedure flawlessly.

Even the best-trained, most conscientious doctors are likely to unintentionally cause harm to their patients occasionally. David Hilfaker in *Healing the Wounds* describes an incident when tests had convinced him that a pregnant patient's baby had died in her womb. The woman and her husband had tried for years to conceive and were very excited. Therefore, it had been especially hard for him to break the bad news to them. Then, while performing a D and C, he realized that he had made a dreadful mistake; the fetus he aborted had been alive. This error was incredibly painful for both Hilfaker and the couple who lost their baby, yet Hilfaker had been convinced he was doing the right thing beforehand. Some doctors might not have admitted their error. Hilfaker did and was forgiven by the couple. In situations like this, when the doctor is doing his best, yet technology provided inaccurate data, I would hope that all patients would have the heart to forgive. Doctors and patients alike must come to terms with the fact that wrong judgments will be made from time to time.

While doctors might not always make the right medical decisions regarding procedures and tests, they *can* develop bedside manners that reassure and instill hope rather than compounding physical pain with additional emotional pain. As mentioned in Chapter 2, patients complain more often about attitudes of physicians than actions. Poor attitudes can cause a great deal of harm—harm that *can* be avoided. Physicians might not even be aware of the pain they inflict because of indifferent attitudes or poor choice of wording. Nevertheless, the end result can in some cases be as detrimental as if that doctor had slipped with the scalpel during surgery.

A patient who feels intimidated or angered by a doctor's manner is less likely to comply with prescribed treatment, less likely to be honest when describing symptoms or behavior, and less likely to return to that doctor when symptoms worsen. I know people who have been so turned off by a physician's attitude they have refused to go back until their conditions have advanced beyond the point of treatment. Patients who don't like a doctor's attitude are also more likely to doctor-shop, which increases the chance of errors as medical records are passed on from one doctor to another. It also increases the overall cost of health care as unnecessary repeat tests are likely to be ordered.

Most patients are forgiving of errors if they like their doctor and feel that he or she is making a best effort to help. Author and nurse Barbara Huttman goes so far as to say that if a patient is fond of his doctor, he is not likely to recognize a "negligent act if it slaps him in the face."[1] Although it is not my goal to encourage unquestioning faith in doctors based entirely on charming bedside manners, a good rapport is a powerful therapeutic tool that can be better used once physicians see how their words and attitudes are likely to impact their patients. Most of the following actions or attitudes that patients frequently protest can easily be remedied when doctors care enough to pay attention to communication skills and choose their words thoughtfully:

1. Patronizing attitudes

While patients do appreciate empathy, most do not want a pat-on-the-head approach from doctors such as "I'm the doctor, let me do the worrying."

Examples of true-life patronizing remarks by doctors:

• To a woman who complained of feeling weak from the neck down: *Oh honey, just blow in a paper bag. You'll be fine.*

Referring to a patient as "honey" is not likely to be taken kindly as it is generally perceived as patronizing or sexist. To be more helpful, he might have discussed hyperventilation as a possibility without being so assuming. He could have taken time to explain how hyperventilation can sometimes cause similar symptoms, perhaps reassuring her that if the paper bag technique didn't help he would consider other possibilities.

• To a married woman who kept her maiden name: *I see you have kept your maiden name. What have you done that is so important?*

This question might simply have been prompted by the doctor's curiosity about this woman's career and perhaps it seemed innocuous to him, but the way it was worded set the tone for a negative encounter and left the patient seething. Again, since it was made by a male to a female patient, it was perceived as sexist and condescending. This woman happens to have a Ph.D. in psychology, but it really shouldn't have mattered. The comment was made by a doctor at a prestigious medical facility, which likely hasn't received any positive endorsements from this woman since.

• To a woman with lupus who was complaining of abdominal pain and digestive problems: *I'm really a smart guy and I can't figure this out. Are you sure you're not bringing this on yourself?*

As discussed earlier, some doctors are quick to blame the patient when answers are elusive.

Irv Anderson, a mechanical engineer, reports that he always dresses in a businesslike manner when he goes to the doctor because he finds that doctors communicate more openly and in a less condescending manner when he does. "When I'm dressed in a suit and tie rather than a sport shirt, doctors treat me more respectfully. They are more open about explaining things and do so on a more technical level. I find this true both on personal visits or when I accompany my wife on her appointments to the Mayo Clinic."

Patients want to be treated as intelligent, responsive human beings. The doctor-patient relationship is moving toward a more balanced interaction with doctors being viewed less as authority figures and more as partners in health care. The very fact that patients traditionally refer to the doctor by title (and doctors seldom encourage otherwise), while the doctor usually refers to the patient by first name, tends to reinforce an authoritarian relationship. It took a long time for me to feel comfortable calling any of the doctors who were involved in my care by their first names, even when I was no longer their patient.

Perhaps encouraging patients to call doctors by first names would result in more balanced communication, although some doctors I discussed this with don't think it is a good idea. Robert Wagner explained that having patients refer to him by his title during office visits was best because of the unique nature of the doctor-patient relationship during which patients often confide quite intimate details about themselves. The title, he said, helped clarify his role as doctor. However, when he stepped outside his "doctor role" he much preferred being called by his first name.

2. Insensitivity

The last thing a patient deserves is to be made to feel foolish about voicing his or her complaints no matter how trivial they seem to the doctor. Yet, this often happens as illustrated by the following examples of remarks that have devastated patients' egos:

• Said with a chuckle to a woman who reported that she was "suffering from low back pain": *You sound like a television commercial.*

This woman confided that she was so humiliated by the doctor's response, she was unable to go on and share any more information about her condition. She left the office feeling belittled and never went back to that doctor.

• To a woman who complained of pain in her elbow (she had seen the doctor on previous occasions, describing pain in her feet and hands): *Oh, you nut!*

This woman was eventually diagnosed with a severe form of degenerative arthritis and has since found a doctor who is compassionate. However, that remark caused her a great deal of anguish and apprehension about seeking help from other doctors. Also a nurse, she suggested that the segment of the Hippocratic oath that says "Physician do no harm" be expanded to say, "Physician do no harm with your mouth."

• To a woman who complained of joint pain: *All women have joint pain—my wife has joint pain, too.*

This woman was, understandably, very put off by this remark. She was eventually diagnosed with lupus. Generalizations like this are very unfair and give the patient no credit for assessing the significance of their own pain, a source of animosity for many.

• To a man who has been diagnosed with fibromyalgia: *What are you dying from today?*

People with disorders that many doctors view as nebulous, such as fibromyalgia and chronic fatigue syndrome, are often treated callously. Physicians whose own families have been touched by these types of illnesses are often the most understanding. After intimate conversations with men and women who suffer from such ailments, I am convinced that the majority of them are suffering a great deal, as their spouses will usually confirm. It is depressing to feel sick and exhausted for months or years on end. When there is so little the medical profession can do for these people, an ounce of compassion seems a small thing to ask and can go a long way in helping the patient cope with symptoms.

• To a young woman who had been dealing with debilitating undiagnosed symptoms for two years: *Go home and bake a pie.*

Although it is understandable that doctors can become

frustrated with patients who appear to have vague illnesses, it isn't fair to the patient to let these attitudes show. From time to time I, too, find myself becoming a bit impatient toward people who call to talk about their illnesses. Then I remind myself how difficult it was for me and how much it meant to hear a kind word or just have someone to talk to, and I vow not to let them down.

Being told "You don't look sick" is also a pet peeve among people who have what Paul J. Donaghue and Mary Siegal describe in *Sick and Tired of Being Sick and Tired* as "invisible chronic illness (ICI)"—illnesses that have few or no objective signs. When a doctor responds to a patient's complaints by telling him he "looks healthy" the patient generally feels the doctor is discounting his symptom report. Therefore, the comment usually invokes anxiety and causes patients to become more focused on symptoms as they wonder how to convince the doctor they are sick.

It is possible for someone to be very ill and in considerable pain, yet look quite well. The week before a friend of mine was hospitalized for her final bedridden days prior to her death from cancer, I heard many people comment on how well she was doing. Some were convinced she was on the mend. And doctors are often no better than lay people at assessing people's health by the way they look. Another friend went to the doctor complaining of chest pain. The doctor ordered an EKG and stress tests before pronouncing him in "great shape." On the way home, the man's chest pain intensified. His wife turned around and headed for a hospital. That very week, at age 42, he underwent open heart surgery during which a triple bypass was performed.

Bonnie Harrison, who has lupus, didn't look sick to her doctor either. She went two years feeling quite ill, forcing herself to continue her full-time job while trying to keep up with a family, before the disorder progressed to serious kidney and liver malfunction which showed up on tests.

Many sick people can shower and groom and pull themselves together long enough to survive a doctor's office visit, yet still have symptoms that are significantly changing the quality of their lives—perhaps making it impossible to work a normal schedule or to get a good night's sleep. Some might have symptoms that never progress to the point of being diagnosable; these people deserve compassion from physicians, perhaps even more so than others because they often do not get much support from family and friends.

One woman confided that a bout with cancer was much less traumatic than fibromyalgia, her current plague. "When I had cancer, friends and family rallied around and were very supportive and encouraging. There were specific medical treatments. No one questioned my mental stability," she explains. "With fibromyalgia, it is the opposite. I am dealing with more physical pain than I ever did from the cancer and there is no help—no compassion from the medical profession and little from others."

When physicians make insensitive comments, the negative impact carries beyond the patient to affect the attitudes of friends and family members toward the entire medical establishment.

Sometimes doctors don't realize their conversations are being held within a patient's hearing range. One of the doctors I saw on many occasions was apparently unaware that one of the exam rooms in his clinic provided no noise insulation. While sitting on the exam table in a scratchy paper gown, I clearly overheard phone conversations about his upcoming ski trips, and about patient cases, including my own. One time he called another physician to discuss my medication and started the conversation with, "I'm calling about you-know-who."

3. Not listening

There is evidence of widespread problems in listening skills among doctors today. Evaluations of routine medical visits showed that doctors retrieved only about 50 percent of information necessary to evaluate patients' conditions. Other studies have shown that physicians cut off patients before they've completely reviewed their symptoms and concerns.[2]

Richard Frankel, a leading expert on doctor-patient communication and co-director of residency training in internal medicine at Highland Hospital in Rochester, New York, found that physicians, on average, gave patients only 18 seconds to describe their medical complaints before interrupting. As a result, the doctors heard only some of the symptoms—and may have missed vital clues.[3]

One study found that between 50 and 90 percent of doctor-patient consultations suffered other kinds of interruptions, such as phone calls, which tended to demolish the patient's concentration.

Doctors who don't listen is indeed a frequent complaint of patients. In my own survey, 50 percent of the respondents said their physicians did not listen. It is frustrating to have waited days, weeks, sometimes even months for an appointment and feel like the doctor is uninterested in hearing what one has to say.

The proliferation of specialists has, in some ways, added to the problem, since they often selectively listen to only the symptoms that seem to fit the realm of their specialty. My own case provides just one example. Because my condition involved choreaform movement, I was referred to a world-renowned neurologist who specialized in movement disorders. Even though I told him that I had a number of what I believed were associated symptoms including joint pain, bladder problems and heart palpitations, he brushed off those symptoms and continued to concern himself only with the movement disorder. Had he paid attention to the other symptoms and considered my instincts that the symptoms were related, it might have occurred to him to include Lyme disease in the differential diagnosis, since chorea as well as all my other symptoms were known symptoms of the disease. During five days of elaborate testing, a test for Lyme was never done, and to my knowledge was not even considered. The doctor concluded I had a "Parkinsonian-type disorder."

Some physicians admit going into specialties to escape the massive uncertainty of the broader field of medicine as well as the tremendous information base given all the new research coming out constantly. Learning a lot about a narrow aspect of medicine can provide a greater sense of security. It can also become a way to escape involvement in ongoing patient care, and too often the specialist becomes narrowly focused.

4. Not spending enough time

After I'd gone through five days of testing at a well known medical clinic, the doctor who was assigned to my case rushed in the door of the consultation room, pulling on his coat as he entered. He sat on the edge of his chair for all of the ten minutes he was there, then rushed out. My husband and I had listened to him hurriedly explain his conclusions regarding my tests not daring to interrupt with questions; we assumed he had a plane to catch. We left feeling disillusioned.

My husband had taken time off work and we had spent hard-earned money to be evaluated by this doctor.

Gale, a Minneapolis woman who has severe rheumatoid arthritis, describes a time when she was scheduled for surgery. After many previous frustrating encounters during which her doctor never stayed in the room long enough to listen to her concerns or answer any questions, she planned a new strategy. The next time her physician rushed in the room she quickly moved her chair in front of the door and sat in it, making it impossible for him to exit before her questions were answered. Evidently, she had a good rapport with this physician and he took it quite well. For her it worked; it jolted him into realizing that she really did need a little more time.

Almost 75 percent of the people I surveyed said that doctors didn't spend enough time with them. And of 1500 people who responded to a poll in *Arthritis Today,* 73 percent of those who claimed to be satisfied with their doctors estimated that their doctors spent at least 10 to 20 minutes with them; only 23 percent were satisfied when their doctors spent 10 minutes or less with them.[+] In fact, in this survey, lack of time spent with the doctor was the most common complaint by those who said they were dissatisfied with overall care. For some, the time problem was further compounded by long waits for the actual visits both in the waiting room and in the exam room.

The data suggests that if more physicians were to spend just a little more time with their patients, overall perceptions of care would improve dramatically. Logic would also suggest that fewer errors would occur.

> *John Witek:* I find that if you take time to talk with the patient, develop some basic trust, you will elicit a significant degree of cooperation from that patient.

While I was his patient, I was in fact amazed at how un-hurried John appeared and how much time he spent on each visit compared to many of the other doctors I had seen. He reinforced that it is not impossible, even in our fast-paced world, for doctors to regulate their schedules to allow patients the time they need to convey their concerns and to get their questions answered. Many of the doctors I interviewed agreed with John that it isn't that difficult to manage schedules to allow an appropriate amount of time for each patient most of the time (although in medical settings where overall income is based on number of patients seen and tests done, some admitted they were pressured by clinic managers to squeeze in more and more patients). St. Paul family practitioner Mary L. Ezzo says that her receptionists are cued to ask patients when they call for an appointment how much time they think they will need. According to internist Laurence Savett, ensuring enough time is primarily a matter of regulating the number of new patients one agrees to see.

Dr. McKegney adds that many physicians are thrown by "schedule-busters"—patients who ask for an appointment to discuss one symptom, then come in with a list of complaints. For instance, a person might ask to be seen for a sore throat and once in the office begin discussing recurring abdominal pain, sex difficulties and problems with weight control. Says McKegney:

> The problem is that most physicians have not been taught they have the right and the obligation to structure the visit without blame or sounding punitive. It is not an easy skill, but it is important to be able to explain to the patient that each of these problems can be addressed, but not necessarily in the same visit.

5. Not explaining things clearly

Too often physicians don't attempt to explain why they are prescribing certain medications or tests. Even when they do, patients who are not familiar with medical jargon can easily become confused.

It is not uncommon for patients to sue when doctors don't take time to explain potential side effects of medications and treatment complications, and the patient suffers a significant problem. I spoke with a man who was livid that his doctor sent him home with the antidepressant amitriptyline with nary a word of advice about the drug. When the patient experienced ringing in the ear and restlessness he procured a pamphlet about the drug from the pharmacist, which not only listed the side effects he had, but warned against operating heavy equipment (which his job normally involved). The doctor would have saved himself much grief had he taken a few minutes to explain these things. Although doctors believe if they talk about side effects the patient will imagine them, or that the patient won't try the medication in the first place, in an age when patients want to be and should be informed, it just isn't a wise policy not to be up front. Except in cases when the patient is incapable of making an informed decision (and then someone else with guardianship powers should be deciding), the legal doctrine of informed consent provides patients the right to decide which risks they want to take. (The doctors' perspective on informed consent is discussed in the next chapter.)

Dr. Stephen Yarnall, a Washington cardiologist, finds it helps to send his patients a written report of what transpired during each visit. When prescribing medication this could be especially helpful.

Although patients must realize it isn't feasible for doctors to know or explain every possible side effect of every medication, when common side effects are discussed beforehand patients aren't as likely to be alarmed if they do occur. John has found it helpful when prescribing a medication to give the patient a pamphlet describing the medication and listing the most common side effects.

His patients are also encouraged to call if they are concerned about other problems that arise after starting the medication.

6. Arrogance

A woman came up to me one day to thank me for writing my second book, saying that it had saved her life. She went on to tell her story:

> I had been dealing with symptoms for nearly two years and was not getting any answers from physicians. I was in pain constantly; I had been forced to quit my job because of fatigue, weakness and neurological symptoms. More than one doctor had suggested MS as a possibility. I asked to be evaluated at [a larger medical facility], hoping to have an MRI since I had been told it could conclusively confirm or rule out MS.
>
> When I inquired about the MRI, the neurologist assigned to my case leaned back, crossed his arms in a cocky manner and asked, "Helen, why do you want to have MS?"
>
> Dumbfounded, I responded, "I don't *want* to have MS. I just want to know what I do have and I was told this test could tell whether or not I have it."
>
> "Well, why do you want to be sick?" he retorted arrogantly.
>
> I had been struggling with depression, primarily because of my illness, and these remarks put me over the edge. I left

the office, got in my car and started driving. I got on the freeway and was driving dangerously fast as I entered the exit ramp. All I could think was that I was going to get home and get a gun and either shoot myself or go back and shoot that doctor. Then suddenly it clicked that I had read a section in your book that mentioned a nurse practitioner that had helped a number of people who had difficult-to-diagnose conditions.

To make a long story short, Helen started weekly sessions with the nurse/counselor who helped her work through a lot of emotional problems as well as connecting her with a medical doctor who had more tolerance for difficult-to-diagnose cases. The nurse started by validating her physical symptoms, reassuring her that she would try to help her get to the bottom of them. Although this woman is still dealing with physical symptoms, she says that emotionally and psychologically she is coping well.

The point of the story is that no one benefits when a physician's manner antagonizes an already distraught patient. If the physician was convinced the MRI would not be helpful, he could have explained why. Perhaps some negotiation could have transpired whereby the doctor agreed to re-evaluate the symptoms several months down the road and then reconsider the possibility of an MRI.

I am convinced that patients will be less likely to insist on expensive tests if their doctors make it clear they will keep an open mind and reevaluate from time to time. My belief is reinforced by interviews with doctors who say their patients are often willing to forgo or delay expensive tests when they take time to explain why those tests aren't likely to be helpful in their situations.

John agrees: A lot of patients come in with ideas about certain tests they want to have done. If I don't feel that the tests they are requesting are likely to provide a clearer picture and explain to them why I don't, I find most patients can understand and accept this.

Dr. Wagner describes his approach:

When patients come in complaining of back pain and asking about an MRI that I may not feel is necessary, I try to help them understand my rationale for choosing not to order one. I ask them whether they feel their condition is bad enough that they are willing to undergo surgery. Most often they say, "Definitely not!" They are much more interested in trying other measures to control the pain. I explain that we can usually get a pretty clear idea of the severity of the condition and location of the injury from a patient's report and the physical exam. Therefore, in the case of chronic back pain, an MRI is usually in order only in cases when pain is so unbearable that surgery is imminent, or the patient is in danger if surgery is not performed.

7. Close-mindedness

Many lay people say they are angered by doctors who are completely close-minded when it comes to treatments not within the realm of conventional medicine. An acquaintance whose young daughter suffered from constant ear infections first consulted a medical doctor. After a year of doctoring during which medications and tubes inserted in the girl's ears failed to provide much relief, the woman decided to try a homeopathic healer. According to her, the homeopath's remedies worked and her daughter no longer has problems with her ears. When she informed the original doctor that she had taken her daughter to a homeopath, he accused her of being a negligent parent. She was so angered by his response that she now refuses to allow a medical doctor to treat any of her family members.

One observer of American medicine writes:

> Of all the mistakes made by physicians that hurt the American people, one of the most powerful and pervasive is their erroneous belief that they alone practice medicine. The truth of the matter is that physicians practice a specific and limited type or school of medical treatment, which uses as its guide a certain belief system they themselves have defined . . . But there are other, nonphysician practitioners, whose belief systems and therapeutic and patient care successes go back as far as the roots of medical establishment history. In fact, some of these practices are at the roots of medical practice . . ."[5]

During college, my sociology professor announced during class one day that he had been diagnosed with lung cancer. He was trying to trust his doctors' treatment recommendations, but had reservations because his experiences with both Western and Indian medicine while serving as a missionary in India had convinced him that Western remedies were not the best choice in every situation. He had witnessed firsthand the success of many of the herbal remedies applied by the native doctors. Their medical knowledge had not come from medical school, but was passed from father to son. One time his young son was bitten by a banana viper, a poisonous snake. On many occasions he had seen the Indian doctors apply their own liquid snake-bite cure, with excellent results. Since there was no Indian doctor in the immediate vicinity at the time, he brought his son for treatment to a doctor who practiced Western medicine. His son's recovery turned out to be slow and complicated. The professor lamented:

The problem I had with the Western doctors is they completely discounted the Indian remedies even though many of them worked very well. The Indian doctors, on the other hand, were open to both Western and Indian remedies.

8. Not caring about the whole person

I have asked many patients, "What could your doctor have done to better help you?" A frequent response was, "He could have acted like he cared" or "She could have seen me as a whole person."

Now we are getting back to the issue of whether doctors have time to address the patient's emotional needs. Clearly, most don't have the time to act as counselors as well as M.D.s. Yet, a few caring words like "I wish I could help you more" or "I know this must be difficult for you" can make the patient feel like he is being seen as a person rather than a disease.

John ended every visit and phone conversation by saying, "Take care"—two simple words that provided a great deal of comfort and made me believe that he did care about me as a person. A few words of kindness from a physician can be a more potent morale booster than from others—perhaps because to the patient he embodies hope for healing.

I recall seeing two different physicians within a few days' time. The first was very abrupt. I came home from the visit feeling let down; my pain seemed overwhelming. The second doctor was kind and explained that although he couldn't offer a diagnosis he would help me find ways to manage the pain. He sent me home with samples of an anti-inflammatory drug, reassuring me that if it didn't help there were plenty of other medications to try. I left the office feeling like my load had been lightened considerably. The medication seemed to help, even though other prescriptions had provided no relief. I was aware at the time that the placebo effect of the caring physician contributed more to the pain management than the drug. His reassurance helped me to relax with the pain, rather than tensing up.

Reporting test results personally, greeting patients in the waiting rooms, calling between visits to see how a patient is doing—people report that these extra touches by physicians mean a great deal.

9. Money-oriented

"They only care about the money" is a common lament among patients about doctors. While I believe the doctors I interviewed who say that most doctors don't choose the profession for the money, the way many fee-for-service clinics are set up, it is hard for some doctors not to become greedy. In these cases, the more patients they see and the more tests performed, the more money they make.

I could almost see the dollar signs in the eyes of one doctor I visited during my illness. He scheduled visits more frequently than even I deemed necessary and seemed very eager to perform repeat tests—and to offer services unrelated to what I was seeing him for, such as gynecological checkups. I continued to see him for a time because he was checking into some possibilities that other doctors had not considered, and I did appreciate that. However, my suspicion that money was his top priority was reinforced one day when he was attempting to insert a long IV catheter into my arm and through my shoulder to my chest. He was having considerable difficulty doing so. After struggling for some time, repeatedly jabbing the needle into my arm and creating a rather bloody mess in the process, he paused in frustration and announced to the nurse standing by, "Boy, I sure am earning my money today!" I was charged over $300 to have the IV inserted. Even with the problems encountered it probably did not take longer than 20 minutes to accomplish the task. The discomfort I experienced wasn't a big deal, but I still felt that he could have pretended to be slightly more concerned about me than about how hard he was working for that $300.

On the other hand, there were doctors who went out of their way to help cut costs and make life easier for me. Rather than scheduling frequent visits, John asked me to call periodically between visits to let him know how I was doing, and occasionally he even made a spontaneous phone call to see how things were going. I always greatly appreciated his willingness to save me the 50-minute trips into the city from our rural home, especially since I wasn't always up to driving myself. I was not charged for any of these phone consultations.

10. Diagnose insensitively

Mark Flapan, Ph.D., describes his experience when diagnosed with scleroderma:

> He [the rheumatologist] asked why I came to see him. I told him about my hands and demonstrated my inability to make a fist. On close inspection, he noted small red spots and indentations on my finger tips and immediately told me I had scleroderma.
>
> Without saying anything more to me he called my doctor to let him know he had diagnosed my case. He seemed more interested in getting recognition for his diagnostic acumen than in telling me anything about my ailment. Whether from his manner or from what he said to my doctor over the phone, I sensed something serious.
>
> After talking to my doctor on the phone, the rheuma-

tologist gave me a thorough examination. When the examination was over, it seemed my "visit" was also over. But something was missing—I was given the name of the disease but wasn't told anything about it. Not only that, I wasn't told what could be done for it.

I needed information; more than that, I needed reassurance. I nervously asked, "What's the treatment for scleroderma?" He matter-of-factly answered, "There's no treatment." I then asked, "What causes it?" He said, "We don't know." I asked, "What's going to happen to me?" He replied with a question, "What do you think?" The question made no sense to me because I didn't know what to think.

Looking back now, I assume this doctor's reticence and evasiveness came out of his discomfort in telling me I had an incurable and life-threatening disease. By saying as little as possible he hoped to avoid upsetting and frightening me. Unfortunately, it didn't work that way.

I would have been spared considerable agony if the doctor who diagnosed my case had given me helpful ways to think about the disease. If he had told me how variable the symptoms and progression of the disease are I would have faced my prospects with less fear. If he had told me that scleroderma is a chronic illness with life-threatening possibilities but not a terminal disease, I would have been less despairing. If he had told me things to do to take care of myself I would have felt less helpless. If he had shown concern for my well-being, I would have felt less alone.[6]

Physicians generally agree that medical school training often does not foster compassionate care. There are many patients who can attest to the unfortunate result.

Before she was diagnosed with lupus, Eileen Radzuinas was hospitalized at a teaching hospital where she was examined by several residents and a medical student. After extensive testing, the medical team returned to her room to report they did not have a clue to the cause of her symptoms. In a book that she wrote about her experience Eileen explains what happened from there:

> Seeing my obvious discomfort as I lowered myself into a seat, they asked where I was hurting, which happened to be my right thigh. I was also experiencing a strong burning sensation in my left arm. They left the room shaking their heads and conferring. I tried to settle into my book, but I was distracted by that terribly disappointing pronouncement [that they didn't know the cause of the symptoms].
>
> I was still staring at the pages of my book when I overheard a conversation that was far more disturbing. For nearly an hour, the voices of these same residents, the medical student, and the senior physician echoed from a nearby hallway into my room. They were reviewing my case. The residents spoke about their frustration . . . They emphasized the severity of my pain and its chronic nature . . . The senior physician's reaction was infuriating beyond words. He downplayed each of the symptoms which were playing havoc with my life . . . The residents interjected at that point to remind him that I was unable to sleep through the night because of the pain. They asserted that I had provided a clear and complete history and that they had found my story convincing . . . The physician interrupted their comments on my behalf and asked them to review the medical information available . . . nothing clinically significant had been found . . . According to him, the best way to make the patient come to terms with the situation is to make her realize that she is not a "medical mystery" . . . He suggested that the most helpful thing for them to do was to tell me that I was perfectly healthy and that I had wasted a lot of time and money on unnecessary testing.
>
> . . . [Later] the medical student came in, and I noticed

the change in his attitude. Unlike the sincere, concerned person he had been earlier, he now acted absolutely pompous. Normally he pulled the curtain to provide some semblance of privacy as we talked. This time he left it wide open, although my roommate had visitors. Within earshot of everyone, he told me that I was a perfectly healthy 35-year-old woman who had wasted a lot of time and money on unnecessary testing. I had to give him credit for having a good memory—he had memorized his supervisor's speech almost verbatim.[7]

About a year later, Eileen's case of lupus was diagnosed based on the results of even more extensive testing, including muscle biopsies and biopsies of the "butterfly" rash that she eventually developed on her face. Ironically, some of the biopsies that revealed gross abnormalities were done at the same teaching hospital where she had been treated so rudely. I wish every medical student, while still impressionable, could read Eileen's compelling book.

I have also had wonderful feedback from medical students and doctors who have read my own story. When doctors and students read and hear real stories from real patients, it helps to counteract the desensitization that often takes place in training. Stories like Eileen's are bound to make an impact, helping young doctors to be more sensitive and keep an open mind as they move into their practices.

6

TOP 10 THINGS THAT
DRIVE DOCTORS CRAZY

There is a real danger in a field that involves such a mixture of art, humanity and science.

— John C. Butler, M.D.

LIKE CHAPTER 5, Patients' Top 10 Complaints About Doctors, the information in this chapter is not based on any formal studies, but has been gleaned from literature written by doctors and from in-depth personal interviews with doctors in a variety of settings and specialties. There are no doubt many more things that drive doctors crazy that aren't addressed in this chapter, but listening to their complaints gave me an enlightening glimpse into their world.

We hear more often of patients' complaints about doctors than we do doctors' complaints about patients and of the many pressures doctors face on a daily basis. I find the more I listen to physicians, the more respectful I am of the challenging role they fill. Although a few said they usually had little trouble leaving their work at the office, others admitted that it was hard to escape the anxiety from the pressures inherent to their profession, including the difficult decisions they make on a daily basis—decisions that are almost always subject to error and run the risk of impacting the well-being of another human being in a negative way. They face enormous challenges—probably more than many of us outside the profession could or would want to handle.

These are the most commonly cited grievances of the physicians who allowed me to temporarily step over the threshold of their world:

1. Patients who don't trust us

The message came through loud and clear that doctors are distraught about the lack of trust from patients. The suspicion and constant questioning of motives were not elements of medicine during the early part of the century. Today, doctors are continually confronted by patients who have their own media-fed beliefs about tests and treatments. John touched on this issue in Chapter 2. Minneapolis internist Gregory Silvis had much to add:

> Patients come in having been coached by [a well-known magazine] on questions to ask me, with the implicit assumption that if they don't watch out for themselves, I am going to exploit them or not have their best interests at heart. When patients come in not trusting, feeling they have to watch their back at every turn, the healing potential in that relationship is far below what could be. It undermines the basic psychological principles of healing. Also, part of the reason it cuts so deeply is that one of my personal neurotic goals for going into medicine was to do good things for people at times they needed it and to have them like me afterward.

I just had a scene recently after prescribing Prozac for a patient with an eating disorder. Prozac is extremely effective in treating eating disorders, not only in comparison to previous antidepressants, but as compared to drugs in general, and is really a very safe drug. Yet people have heard otherwise from some of the media, so I am often questioned when I prescribe it. This particular patient was struggling a lot with obsessional thoughts about food and, from experience, I was convinced she could be helped by Prozac, and therefore recommended it. It was clear the family was uncomfortable about it, so I asked them to talk about their feelings. The mother responded indignantly, "Well! I just know that Prozac is a very dangerous drug! I saw this doctor on Oprah Winfrey and he said doctors are prescribing it all the time and don't know what they're doing—it's just very dangerous!"

There was this sort of assumption that if she didn't watch out for her daughter I was going to *get* her—that I didn't have her daughter's best interests at heart, but rather was going to benefit in some ill-defined way by putting her on Prozac. Not only that—by watching a 15-minute Oprah segment she assumed that she could know as much about prescribing Prozac as I did.

I confess that I didn't handle this situation very well. I ended up sort of belittling the woman by saying, "Gee, I wonder why Oprah is on the air. I wonder if she is there to convey medical information or to sell soap."

I'm thankful that we have talked more since then, and I feel we have managed to patch things up.

As John also mentioned previously, some of the mistrust among patients is motivated by their impression that insurance companies seem to have considerable input regarding their care (or attempt to). Therefore, when a doctor opts not to do a particular test or treatment, patients might suspect that she is basing her decision on the wishes of the insurance company, rather than what she truly believes is in the patient's best interests.

2. List-carrying patients

I had become aware of the negative impressions that some physicians have toward patients with lists before I started this book, but was surprised at the degree of stress that lists cause many of them. This was the first issue that one doctor addressed when I posed the question: What is most frustrating to physicians about patients?

Although some doctors make a point of asking their patients to keep records and lists of symptoms to bring to follow-up visits, my research into this issue has revealed that, in general, patients who come to doctors' offices with unsolicited lists are more likely than not to create barriers to developing a positive rapport. They also run a much greater risk of being labeled neurotic.

Doctors had a lot to say about list-writers—so much that I had enough material to write a separate chapter on this topic. To learn more about how doctors react to list-carrying patients see Chapter 7.

3. Patients who pressure us to make diagnoses or prescribe treatments

Because many people don't understand the diagnostic process very well and have gross misperceptions about the fallibility of medical technology, they don't realize that diagnosing a problem might take considerable time and that, even when a diagnosis can be made, many conditions do not have specific cures or treatments. Finding the right approach to managing symptoms might involve a long process of trial and error.

> *John Witek:* The attitude of many patients today is "Why can't you just tell me what's wrong?" We wind up spending a significant amount of time dealing with vague symptoms for which patients want definitive answers right away. Other patients aren't happy unless we say what they are expecting to hear.

"It is hard when we try to do what we feel is right, yet patients respond with anger no matter what you do," says Yarnall who told the following story:

> One of my patients, a woman in her nineties, has severe arthritis. I prescribed some pretty strong medication to ease her severe pain, warning her not to take too much. She finished the prescription rather quickly, then called asking me to refill the prescription by phone. I really don't like to do this, but I finally succumbed to her pressuring and called in a second prescription. Again, she used up the medication and called back asking for a refill. When I refused, telling her that I'd like her to make an appointment to see me so we could reevaluate the situation, her son got on the phone and became hostile, accusing me of being money-hungry. Again I gave in and prescribed the medication. Then, after she wound up having a big GI bleed, I was accused of not warning her of the dangers of the medication—yet, I had warned her. I was only trying my best to help. It isn't pleasant when people are angry no matter what you do.

Because the mindset of many patients is that pills will fix their problems, it can be hard to convince them that a prescription is not in order, says Mary Ezzo:

> I won't prescribe drugs unless they are needed, but it is often hard to convince patients that it is not in their best

interests to do so. Although some of my patients have a more holistic attitude and appreciate my position on this, more often patients are disappointed when I don't give them something to take home. I've made it a habit to provide them educational material whenever possible so they do have something in hand when they leave the office, which seems to help.

4. Patients who seem to cultivate illness

One doctor lamented:

> Some people seem to take great pride in having complex medical problems and listing the number of times they have been hospitalized or operations they have had. These patients demand a tremendous amount of time and energy and aren't very pleasant to work with. They seem to enjoy spending time in doctors' offices and making a big show out of their conditions.

Doctors agree that it is much more pleasant for physicians to deal with patients who are more focused on the positive than on the negative.

5. Patients with entitlement mentalities

Many doctors see a general unwillingness among people to assume any responsibility for their health; too much of the responsibility, they say, is placed in the hands of the physician. "People don't take care of themselves, then expect the doctor to fix everything," says Wagner:

> I see patients who are abusing their bodies by eating all the wrong things or indulging in excessive amounts of alcohol, yet refusing to change their behavior. They then come expecting me to fix their hypertension; it is aggravating.

I see the patient as the primary manager of his or her life. Ideally, a patient should come to me regarding a specific issue and my role is to act as a consultant, drawing from what I have learned in medical school and from my experiences as a physician. The patient is ultimately responsible for deciding whether to take the services or advice I offer, then to go on managing his life.

John Butler agrees:

Some patients have the notion that I am responsible for fixing everything. Especially in this country, people have the notion they aren't responsible for any of their ailments. I have practiced in Thailand and England and have noticed that this entitlement mentality is more prevalent here than elsewhere. People refuse to see any connection between their bad habits—smoking, lack of exercise, poor eating habits—and their health. They expect someone else to take care of them—they want me to treat everything for them.

John Witek adds:

Some people are quick to call doctors for relatively minor problems. They will call the physician's office and insist on being seen as soon as possible, and by the time they arrive, their symptoms have already cleared up.

Advice on knowing when to call the doctor is probably best obtained from one's own doctor. It will depend on a patient's particular situation. Many clinics provide telephone access to a nurse who can offer basic medical information that is helpful in making a decision.

6. The money issue

I had not considered discussing money issues when I first started writing this book, but the subject was brought up several times during my interviews with doctors, and I realized that for many it is a source of consternation.

Doctors are angry about being accused of being money-hungry as if they alone are to blame for high health care costs. In fact, the cost of health care is complex and the medical professional is only one of many players. Technological and pharmaceutical advances bring new costs. Litigation is a factor, as is the insurance establishment, including how consumers use their insurance.

While a large assortment of corporate management types, entertainers and others enjoy impressive "market value" with little public outcry, many people are quick to complain about the bill from the doctor, perhaps because it seems to affect them more directly—and they may not entirely understand just what it was they got for their money.

7. Media-generated hysteria

Doctors cringe every time the media dramatically portrays "the disease of the month" for they know their phone lines will be flooded and their offices will be packed with people they will be hard-pressed to convince probably don't have the disease. More distressing are diagnosed patients whose hopes for cures are falsely raised by media hype. Many media reports of new tests, treatments or cures are based on preliminary or early research, usually on limited numbers of patients. The truth becomes more apparent as more are evaluated.

Finding a balance and keeping an open mind in such situations can be difficult. The fact that I am a former Lyme patient has made it somewhat more of a challenge to gain trust from some physicians, since many of them are defensive about what they view as Lyme hysteria caused by massive publicity. The fact that I wrote about my experiences with the disease has compounded the problem causing some to accuse me of adding to this hysteria. The truth is that at the time I began writing about my experiences I didn't know I had Lyme disease or that the disease would become such big news for so many years.

8. Outside forces

Aside from complaints about patients, doctors had complaints about outside forces that sometimes seem to dictate the way they practice. As health care has become more high tech and more costly in this country, and people have become more dependent on the medical profession to prevent and resolve their health problems, insurance companies and government agencies have become an integral part of the health care process. Although most would agree that our health care system could not function without their involvement, it makes medical practice more complex and significantly impacts the doctor-patient relationship.

Some doctors say they feel they are seen as adversaries by both the patients and the insurance companies. "It is almost impossible to avoid conflicts," says Yarnall. "The doctor-patient relationship was already wounded. Now it is incredibly threatened by outside forces—many of which are neither the doctor's nor the patients' fault."

Along with the involvement of insurance companies and government agencies has come an enormous amount of bureaucracy and added paperwork. Doctors complain about needing to justify many of their decisions with these outside forces.

Keeping up with disability and workers' compensation forms can be particularly cumbersome, according to John:

I understand the necessity of forms to keep insurance companies updated on a patient's status and to help keep people honest. But there are times that I am continually asked to fill out forms on specific patients when there seems to be no rationale for doing so. I have a patient with Huntington's chorea and have pointed out many times on the forms I've sent back that this is a progressive, hereditary, neurological disease which the patient will eventually die from. This patient cannot work and, barring a miracle from God, he will continue getting worse. Yet, the insurance company continues to send me forms to fill out every month, asking "How has he been?" and "Is there any chance for improvement?" If someone has a back problem, I can see why they might continue to question it, but cases like this make no sense.

It is also frustrating, according to Mary Ezzo, when people don't take responsibility for understanding their medical insurance polices:

The very hardest part of my job is that my patients are covered by a lot of different insurance companies whose policies regarding coverage vary considerably. Many of my patients are penalized if they don't use certain hospitals or clinics. Just recently I saw a patient for a pre-op consultation who was scheduled for surgery the next morning. However, when I called for clearance from her insurance company I learned that she was not covered at the surgical center where it was to take place.

We can't possibly keep track of which companies cover what and where. It takes a lot of time that could be spent taking care of people.

Doctors complain that it is more difficult to act in what they feel are the best interests of their patients, or to do what patients expect them do. Silvis describes two world views of medicine: "One is about trust, partnerships and compassion;

the other is an adversarial view aggravated by legal intrusions into the profession."

Doctors are expected to make the medical decisions, while someone else makes the economic decisions. Doctors are the ones liable for outcomes, yet they are faced with obstacles when it comes to acting in what they feel are their patients' best interests. Silvis said the following scenario is not uncommon:

> I might want to admit a patient to the hospital late in the afternoon on a Friday. I call the insurance company to make sure they'll pay for it. They tell me the office is closed till Monday. It becomes my decision to admit the patient or not, but I won't know until Monday if the insurance company is going to pay for it.

Obviously, these situations create a dilemma for doctors. If the doctor decides not to admit the patient and that patient turns out to have more serious problems because of it, the doctor could be blamed for negligence. But if the doctor decides to admit the patient, the insurance company will typically review the decision, and if it deems the case not serious enough to warrant admission it may refuse payment, and the patient is likely to be angry about that as well.

Silvis adds:

> On the other hand, if I tell families that from past experience I am sure an insurance company won't pay for a test or procedure, and I don't think it's even going to be worth going to them, I become the bad guy. It is very uncomfortable.

9. Pressures and lack of freedom

Some are just angry about the pressure and lack of freedom the job allows. As Wagner says:

You put your heart and soul for years into training, expecting that it will give you some freedom. But, you find there is really no freedom at all. You are in service to patients, colleagues, nursing staff, and your own ideals. The pressures and responsibilities can be enormous. Doctors often feel trapped. The proverbial buck always stops with the doctor.

When you look at it historically, the legislature assigned doctors to be the ones who prescribe the drugs, do the invasive things. The AMA deliberately worked to channel control toward doctors so they could collect fees for these things. In the long run this has worked terribly against us. So much extraneous stuff comes to the doctor. We are the victims of our own lobbying efforts in a sense.

10. Informed consent

The doctrine of informed consent, which is about 25 years old in this country, provides patients the right to be informed about risks of tests and treatments prescribed by doctors and to make the decisions regarding their own care.

Although doctors agree that in theory informed consent is good, many see it as an obstacle to developing a positive rapport with their patients.

> *John Witek:* I think it creates a different attitude in the doctor-patient relationship—a more cautious, less smooth relationship. A physician should be able to function as a patient advocate, helping patients navigate their way through medical science, making suggestions while explaining all the options. The doctrine of informed consent causes you to move out of the patient advocate role, to think in legal terms. You become concerned with covering your own tail by making sure you've told the patient virtually everything that could go wrong, when the chances are they will go right.

While patients should know what they are getting into and be informed about the chances for good and bad outcomes of treatments and procedures, it can be difficult for people who are not trained scientifically or who do not have a good understanding of statistics to really comprehend what it means when a doctor starts talking about risk percentages. Once you start mentioning risks, even if they are remote, people tend to focus on the negative. For instance, studies have shown the drug tacrine (Cognex) to be somewhat effective in combating the memory loss of Alzheimer's disease, and I agreed to be involved in an ongoing trial use of this drug. However, there were a lot of things to explain to patients about the drug. After I discussed the potential side effects with my patients, not a single one wanted to sign up to try it.

People tend to have naive beliefs about what medicine can do; they deny any of the negatives and expect to get treatments with no side effects. Yet, there is no drug that exists that doesn't have potentially negative effects.

Even though the concept of informed consent is good, it is difficult to get truly informed consent from most people. There is no way to standardize it. You can only get *more informed* consent, and most people still accept treatments based on their faith in the physician who offers them. No matter how you try to explain risks to patients, attorneys probably can find ways to tear apart your explanations.

7

THE LIST-CARRYING
PATIENT

I HAVE before me an article from a reputable magazine. The article, about doctor-patient communication, offers a number of suggestions for those who want to be sure they get the most out of their doctor visits. Typical of such articles, this one recommends bringing a written list of symptoms and questions to ask the doctor. The advice is good, but far too often the articles fail to mention a key point: The written list can create more problems for the patient than it solves if it is not employed in a sensitive manner.

I would never have known this had I not run across the following bit of information several years ago in a book by Larrian Gillespie, M.D. She says:

> It seems that many physicians have been taught to beware of patients carrying lists because list makers have a reputation for being phobic. It is not known where this stereo-

type originated but recently a family practitioner from Alabama, Dr. John F. Burnum, debunked it in the prestigious *New England Journal of Medicine.* The *Journal* rarely runs nonscientific articles, but Dr. Burnum's article was anecdotal, based on his own observation that list-writing patients were quite sane. The editors believed the subject extremely important and thus ran the article as a way of alerting physicians to this point of view.

"Traditional medical wisdom holds that patients who relate their complaints to their physicians from lists are, ipso facto, emotionally ill," Dr. Burnum wrote. "DeGowin and DeGowin in their venerable textbook on diagnosis say that note writing is 'almost a sure sign of psychoneurosis. The patient with organic disease does not require references to written notes to give the essence of his story.'" [1]

Gillespie reports Burnum's observations of seventy-two list-writing patients of whom he found most to be emotionally stable:

> Almost all of these emotionally normal list writers had serious physical disorders . . . Patients with organic disorders, therefore, do refer to written notes to give the essence of their story—and not because they are peculiar or crazy.[2]

No doubt lists can help people recall questions they want to ask and symptoms they want to discuss. A personal journal might reveal symptom patterns which could provide clues to a diagnosis. But are lists and journals likely to enhance rapport between patient and doctor? It depends on how they are used. An unsolicited list or journal produced by the patient is likely to have a negative effect. It's important that doctor and patient together establish the need and purpose of such records if they are to be used productively.

In the years since I read Dr. Gillespie's book I have questioned dozens of doctors about "the list" and the majority of them have confirmed, some more cautiously than others, that lists often antagonize doctors and are more likely than not to create a wall of discomfort between the doctor and patient, especially if they are brought on the first visit.

Dr. Robert Wagner was most candid about this issue going so far as to reveal a passionate distaste among fellow physicians for list-carrying patients that is almost universal in his estimation: "A patient with a list in hand almost invariably rouses anger in physicians—some react to them so intensely they come close to hyperventilating when confronted by a list-carrying patient."

Wagner's revelation validated the experiences of patients who shared with me doctors' reactions to their own lists. None of them realized at the time what had prompted the abrupt changes in their doctor's behavior—some claimed doctors who were previously quite amiable suddenly seemed agitated and hostile.

Unfortunately, patients who have the most trouble finding compassionate physicians in the first place—those with ongoing undiagnosed symptoms—are probably most likely to resort to lists believing that it will help them remember things they might have forgotten to report earlier—things they hope might turn up a clue that will solve their medical mysteries.

Only one time during the six-plus years that I searched for a diagnosis did I bring a list to a doctor visit. I'm almost embarrassed to admit now that it was a full notebook-sized sheet of paper itemizing even some incidents that had occurred while I was a youngster and teenager. What made me decide to bring a list this time—more than five years into my illness? Several family members had literally hounded me to do so for some time. They were convinced that the reason the doctors weren't diagnosing me was that I wasn't providing enough information. "Did you ever tell them about the fainting spell you had in 1969? What about the frequent headaches that you had back in . . .?" they asked over and over.

On this particular visit I was scheduled to see a neurologist on a referral. I knew this was a one-time visit and this doctor supposedly had some expertise in movement disorders. This time I was determined to take full advantage of the visit and tell her everything—I would leave no stone unturned that might have a remote chance of relating to my current medical dilemma—just in case.

Needless to say, the doctor was clearly annoyed with me from the outset; I soon realized that she wasn't the least bit interested in knowing what was on my list, and I sensed that she could not wait to get me out the door and go on to the next patient. Like others with similar stories, at the time I was only vaguely aware of the impact of my list on her attitude toward me. I now realize that it was likely significant. It would be interesting to replay the encounter minus the list.

While speaking at a chronic illness support group meeting recently, I brought up the list issue. One woman commented that she always brings a list and wondered if that might be why her doctor refers to her as one of his "most difficult patients." Another woman claimed that her doctor changed his diagnosis from a physical one to a psychological one when she brought a list along to her appointment.

Dr. Wagner admits that doctors' reactions to lists are irrational but are also ingrained:

> There may be a few doctors who have matured enough to have gone beyond feeling hostile about patient lists and are able to view them as simply a practical reminder. After all,

we take shopping lists to the grocery store, why shouldn't we take lists to the doctor's office? However, more often the physician's immediate response is: This patient is going to take a lot more time; I'm going to get behind!

There is also the issue of control. Those who go into the profession tend to like control; we are self-starters, are relatively independent thinkers, have well developed egos, are compulsive, and perfectionistic. In fact, MMPIs taken by physicians often indicate slight aberrations in these areas. We are then further conditioned by our training to be in control. The patient with the list turns the tables; he or she gains control of the interview. The doctor's agenda is disrupted; he can no longer proceed in the orderly manner to which he is accustomed.

In some ways the list also becomes a barrier to developing the relationship between the doctor and patient which is so important. The physician's job can only be done well in the context of a good relationship. It seems harder to relate directly to each other in a personal way when a list is involved.

Dr. Butler agrees that physicians often feel overwhelmed when a patient comes with a list of complaints as it might mean he will be confronted with ten different problems— and he feels he has to deal with them all immediately. "The task becomes so large that it can't possibly be accomplished in one visit," he adds. As another doctor put it, "When I see a list, I think of it as a 'schedule-wrecker.' I'm going to have to deal with a whole list of complaints in a time slot in which I would normally deal with just one."

When I questioned one doctor about lists, she initially had nothing but good things to say. Lists, she said, helped reveal what was on her patients' minds and helped her get to the point in answering their questions. However, when I mentioned a list on the first visit, her attitude changed completely:

When patients bring a list on the first visit I view them as doctor shoppers. I don't think it's appropriate to bring a list on the first visit. It creates an unequal relationship from the start; it doesn't give me an opportunity to get to know the patient. I don't see myself as the right doctor for that kind of patient.

Of all the physicians who talked about lists, Cate McKegney was the most consistently positive:

I don't mind lists. In fact, I kind of like it when patients bring them. I like them because at least I know what I am dealing with. Some people come in with an agenda in their head and it's a lot harder to negotiate about that than about something that is written down. When there's a piece of paper, we can talk about what's on it and about what's realistic to expect on the visit.

My response to a list is not to say, "Oh good, we're going to deal with all those things today." When somebody comes in with a list that involves every major organ system, I usually say, "There are a lot of things here and we need to attend to them appropriately. Which two do you want to discuss today?" I explain that we'll get to all the items on the list eventually and add, "You and I are going to figure out a plan about how to handle this. It might mean having you come in once or perhaps twice a week for the next month."

It's kind of like writing a book. We can't write all the chapters simultaneously. We write them one at a time and, once all ten are written, we might find that one goes with a different book.

Most people come in expecting a lot of things from me; when they aren't written down it's a lot harder to talk about them. I've been fortunate to have been taught the skills on how to negotiate the patient's agenda, but most physicians haven't. Most of them have been taught by physicians who say if you see a list, you're in big trouble. You're not in big trouble; you're just in a different kind of trouble in the sense that you have a different kind of task. The first task is going to be to say more explicitly, "Gosh, there are a lot of things you're expecting from me." But, at least you can say it.

A list—who would have thought something so small and seemingly innocuous could cause so much tension, bewilderment, and misunderstanding? The list-carrying patient is a prime example of a situation in which the doctor-patient encounter often fails to be effective because one or the other is ignorant of the other's agenda; it illustrates why it is so important for doctors and patients to be honest with each other. If patients and doctors can discuss this issue more openly, it should be possible to minimize the frustration of lists for both.

John's approach might be helpful for others:

The list is not a bad idea if it is used effectively. In fact, if a patient comes in without a list and can't coherently recite their story—perhaps hems and haws about the timing and sequence of events—it is frustrating for both of us.

On the other hand, there really isn't time to read a long narrative. When someone brings in a multi-page list with writing so small even they can't read it, it is not in any way helpful—and I have to admit it makes me a bit anxious. In those situations, I try to take the bull by the horns and explain that I am not going to be able to deal with everything on the list during that visit. I suggest that they start with the most important issues, and we'll deal with those first. Some of the less important problems might have to be dealt with on a later visit. If they have a complicated history, I also suggest they highlight key words and symptoms to make it easier to do a quick review of the list, or that they use cue cards rather than a list to help them remember important points. I sometimes tell patients to write down what's happening between visits, but when I do, I try to give some guidance to make it more effective.

The list might be a bigger issue for primary care physicians who often slot shorter amounts of time for each patient. Ideally, patients should be aware of the amount of time scheduled for their visit. If a patient is only scheduled for 15 minutes, a long list will be more disconcerting for the doctor, who will probably start thinking about the other patients yet lined up in the waiting room—patients who will probably be angry by the time he gets around to them because of the delay. The patient who has a lot to discuss might have to ask to be scheduled for a longer appointment.

One doctor's comment about lists was, "If a patient's symptoms are so mild that he needs to write them down in order to remember them, then it seems like those symptoms aren't very significant anyway." I realized from his statement that some physicians don't have a very good understanding of the reasons patients write lists. Therefore, I thought it might be helpful to "list" some of the many reasons that people bring lists to doctors' offices.

PATIENTS' REASONS FOR BRINGING LISTS

• *They are nervous about the visit, which makes it hard to remember questions they want to ask.* Even normally confident, well-educated people admit feeling very nervous about being in a doctor's office and, once there, they often sense the doctor is in a hurry. Therefore, even if they have only a few questions they want to be sure to have answered, past experience has proven they usually forget to ask one or more them.

• *It is difficult to remember the timing and sequence of events.* Doctors almost invariably ask how long symptoms have been going on, and it is often difficult to remember off the top of one's head. Also, people might have several symptoms but are unsure if any of them are related. Writing down the details of symptoms, including when they started in relation to each other, seems logical.

• *They can't remember names and dosages of medications.* Older people, especially, often have trouble remembering what medications and specific dosages they are taking—again, these are details that are important for the physician to know.

• *They are told to do so.* Sometimes physicians ask people to keep a record of events between visits. However, even more often the patient has read numerous articles about "making the most out of your doctor visit," advising that a list is one key to a productive visit.

• *They are obsessive.* There are, no doubt, some true hypochondriacs who are obsessed with symptoms, and some people with organic diseases might be as well. In fact, when one has a long-undiagnosed illness, it is easy to become somewhat preoccupied with symptoms.

John suggests, if patients do bring a list, to make it just a brief list of key points to use as a reminder. Another solution for the patient is to write down everything she wants to ask or tell the doctor and tuck the list into a pocket or purse. Just writing it down will help in remembering, and reviewing it in the waiting room will help in recalling anything that has been forgotten. In fact, one study showed patients who wrote down and reviewed their thoughts while sitting in doctors' waiting rooms asked doctors more relevant questions and, afterward, felt more in control of their situation.[3]

8

MISCOMMUNICATION

LIST-CARRYING patients aside, there are a number of other factors conducive to misunderstandings between doctors and patients. Sometimes well-intentioned attempts to communicate information go awry. It should be helpful for both parties to be aware of some factors that can contribute to miscommunication:

What seems good news to the physician might seem bad news to the patient

There are times when doctors and patients fail to communicate very well because they view situations from opposite perspectives. For instance, a patient study at London Hospital Medical College demonstrated that doctors often relay information to a patient assuming that it will help calm anxieties and fears when in reality it is received in the opposite light. Hoping to reassure patients and give them a positive outlook, they routinely told patients their diseases were mild and in the early stages:

> Compared with other patients, this was often the case, but for individual patients it did not make sense. In their terms they were in considerable pain, might have had deformities and feared for the future. The idea that this was the "mild" form of the disease or in its early stages merely heightened their anxieties and fears for the future—the opposite of what was intended. It often caused the patient to think—If this is mild, how am I going to manage if it gets worse? [1]

Depending on the disease, perhaps it would be more helpful for physicians to explain that not all patients with a particular disease get progressively worse, that some do get better over time. In fact, many chronic illnesses are unpredictable and may have a propensity to go into remission for long periods of time, sometimes permanently.

A second situation in which differing mindsets between doctor and patient often causes misunderstandings was described in the first chapter in the Bob Stephens scenario. Doctors generally expect patients to indicate relief when test results come back normal. Yet, depending on the nature and duration of symptoms, the patient might actually be disappointed, since to them it might simply mean the tests are missing something. I recall coming home from many a doctor visit feeling incredibly discouraged for having spent so much time in doctors' offices and money on tests only to learn once again that I was no closer to answers than when I started. When a patient seems disappointed that tests are normal, I fear that doctors frequently misconstrue the reaction as a desire to be sick.

People are often greatly relieved to be given a diagnosis,

even when the disease is serious and the prognosis poor. Once that diagnosis sinks in they might go through an adjustment period, but the initial reaction is almost invariably a sense of relief about being freed from the limbo of "not knowing." Dr. Savett confirms that while people have difficulty dealing with uncertainty, most ultimately learn to handle the news of a serious disease:

> The known is much easier to accept than the unknown. People accept bad news all the time, and they accept it very well. Beyond that, a serious diagnosis causes people to recognize their own mortality and the preciousness of time, and it often becomes an especially meaningful time in their lives.

When an illness is life-disrupting, the longer the symptoms have gone unnamed, the happier the person is likely to be about getting the diagnosis. I'll never forget the exhilaration I felt walking out of the doctor's office after being given an official diagnosis of Lyme disease, even though the doctor told me that some of my symptoms might be permanent and that there was a good chance that I would relapse. Fortunately, I never did relapse—my symptoms continually improved following treatment and today, over seven years later, I am virtually free of Lyme disease symptoms. However, even if I had not done so well, having a diagnosis to rest on would have made my life and the lives of my family members easier in many ways.

In my previous book I shared the story of a man from my home town who had symptoms of a brain tumor that took about a year for doctors to diagnose. When doctors were finding "nothing wrong," his wife says he vowed to her many times he would never complain again if someone could just find what was wrong. She reported that from the time he was told he had a brain tumor until he died nine months later, he kept that promise.[2] This man found it easier to cope with the known—even though it meant he was dying from a brain tumor—than to deal with disturbing symptoms of an unknown cause.

Doctors tend to think in probabilities while patients think in possibilities

When it comes to ordering tests, a doctor's past experience along with what she has read will greatly influence her decisions about when to order them. John Butler explained that if a physician's knowledge, biomedical training, and experience dictate that the probability of a patient having a certain problem is very low, she isn't likely to think it appropriate to order expensive tests to look for it. Costs of medical care are already out of control, and it just isn't feasible to put every patient who walks in the door through an elaborate series of tests. According to Dr. Ronald D. Franks, Dean of the University of Minnesota Medical School, Duluth, it costs between $100,000 and $1 million dollars to diagnose a brain tumor today (taking into consideration that, according to one radiologist, one MRI in a thousand detects a brain tumor). To complicate the decision making, even the most sophisticated tests produce results that have to be interpreted on a case by case basis. Therefore, performing a test does not necessarily help clarify the diagnosis or the best approach to treatment in any given situation, says Butler:

> There are large gray areas when it comes to evaluating medical tests. People just don't realize that tests will sometimes show abnormalities even when a person is healthy. For instance, a stress test might show some irregularities in a person who has a very healthy heart. Therefore, even when we strongly suspect there is no serious problem, once

the test has been done, we are forced to pursue it even further—perhaps do more invasive testing that might not be at all to the patient's benefit. [It is also possible for test results to appear normal when there are actually significant abnormalities. No test is perfect.]

While physicians tend to focus on probabilities, patients tend to focus on possibilities. Patients tend to assume that if a medical test is available, it is always appropriate to use it. If there is any possibility that a serious problem exists, they want it checked out thoroughly using the most sophisticated tests available. As Dr. Silvis says, from the patient's perspective there is no such thing as good enough in medicine. They might undergo a test with a 90 percent probability of finding a problem that shows nothing amiss. Yet, if they hear of another test with a 95 percent probability of finding that problem, they want that test done too.

These two opposing mindsets often make for friction between doctors and patients. At times it becomes necessary to compromise. If a patient's symptoms are validated by the doctor, and that doctor reassures her that he is going to continue to work with her on finding solutions, she may be more likely to accept postponement of expensive, risky, or inconclusive medical tests until there is further evidence that they will be useful.

Patients who intentionally provide unreliable information out of fear

When a patient provides inconsistent or unreliable information it can drive doctors a bit crazy, but perhaps it will be helpful for doctors to understand some of the reasons this happens and for patients to understand why it is best to be honest. The following story shared by a friend concerns an optometrist visit, but the problem is frequently encountered in other medical settings as well:

> My 73-year-old mother had been complaining for some time about vision problems. She had visited several optometrists and each time came away upset that a stronger glasses prescription, which seemed to her the only logical solution, had not been forthcoming. Finally, I agreed to accompany her on a visit. It was enlightening. As I observed the optometrist performing the eye exam, I realized my mother was responding to his questions in a manner she thought would convince him she needed stronger glasses, not in a manner consistent with what she was actually seeing. This, of course, was only frustrating the doctor and skewing the test results.
>
> After completing the exam, the optometrist tried to explain to my mother that her vision problems were caused by cataracts, a problem that stronger glasses would not correct. He suggested surgery as a possibility and recommended she see an ophthalmologist. My mother was nodding as if she understood what he was saying, but I knew her well enough to realize it was not sinking in. Since I have talked to her all my life, I felt I was able to explain the problem to her in a manner that was easier for her to grasp. I was also able to explain to the optometrist why my mother was being so inconsistent in her responses to the questions he asked during the eye exam. He felt better knowing that family members could understand his frustration and didn't fault him for the predicament.

In my friend's mother's case, having a third party involved helped. Especially when dealing with the elderly, it might be a good idea to encourage a close friend or family member to sit in on a visit to assess the situation when it is clear that there is a communication problem.

Like the woman who gave inconsistent responses to the optometrist's questions during her eye exam, it is not unusual for patients to hesitate to be completely honest with doctors out of fear they won't be believed or helped if they are. Sometimes they are confused by their symptoms. The way symptoms are behaving might not seem logical, and they fear candidness will convict them as "crazy." They may, in fact, be questioning their own sanity despite their instincts to the contrary. For instance, although many illnesses cause symptoms that come and go or fluctuate in intensity, more than one person has confided to me their fear of reporting these symptom irregularities to their physicians. To those who don't understand that the nature of many illnesses is to produce day to day changes, these fluctuations in symptom intensity don't make sense.

Again I can pull an example from personal experience. About two years into my illness, I developed an involuntary choreaform movement. After 30-some years of being accustomed to deciding how and when my muscles and limbs would move, they suddenly seemed to have a will of their own. Past experience dictated that I should be able to stop the jerking muscle movement. However, although I could sometimes momentarily restrain the movement by concentrating very hard, this only caused it to burst forth with even more intensity as soon as I let my guard down. During flare-ups, the movement continued for weeks or months nonstop during waking hours. When I slept it was quiet, and sometimes even during the day it was relatively subdued. However, whenever I was around other people, or when there was a lot of visual and auditory stimuli, it was more pronounced. Attending one of my children's band concerts or joining friends in laughter invariably put it in high gear.

Initially, I didn't report these observations to doctors. It came as a great relief when John volunteered that certain stimuli will temporarily aggravate any movement disorder, adding that his Parkinson's disease patients complain that their tremor often acts up much more when they are out and about than when they are at home. He explained that it is normal for movement disorders to be calmed during sleep.

Unfortunately, while many patients are not completely honest amidst the confusion and fear, I now realize that not reporting symptoms accurately is likely to diminish their credibility with doctors. Therefore, I do encourage patients to share all observations about their symptoms.

Patients find it difficult to describe symptoms

Patients often struggle to find the right words to describe their conditions. When they can't find a way to put their discomfort into words—when they are vague about where symptoms are located or how often they occur—doctors are less likely to take them seriously.

Unfortunately, a patient who is experiencing numerous symptoms (which is often the case with lupus, Lyme disease and many other diseases, including many neurological diseases) may be quite uncertain about which symptoms are significant. Once the patient really starts to feel ill, it is easy to start recalling previous incidences of milder symptoms and wonder if those, too, are in some way related and might offer clues. Thus patients often come in with what physicians view as an inordinately long litany of symptoms.

It would be helpful if a physician could just experience the patient's symptoms for a moment or two. Since this is impossible, attempting to explain symptoms so that doctors can understand is likely to always be a challenge.

Patients misinterpret doctor's explanations

Sometimes a doctor is certain that a patient understands the information presented to him when that patient has, in reality, completely misconstrued it. A good example occurred a few years ago. I received a phone call from a woman I'll call Sandy who had a possible case of Lyme disease. She had been prescribed antibiotics by one doctor, which had temporarily improved her condition. However, when the symptoms returned a few months later, the doctor refused to treat her with another round of antibiotics.

She then consulted Dr. D., whom I know quite well. He generally has an excellent rapport with his patients and is very conscientious about taking time to offer explanations for his decisions and conclusions. Shortly after her consultation with Dr. D., Sandy phoned the leader of a local Lyme disease support group complaining that when she asked Dr. D. about the possibility that she had experienced a Jarisch-Herxheimer reaction he had told her there is no such thing. (A Jarisch-Herxheimer reaction describes a temporary worsening of symptoms, usually fever and chills, after starting antibiotic therapy.) The support group leader, who knew that I was a friend of Dr. D.'s, relayed this information to me. Finding it hard to believe that Dr. D. would tell her something I knew to be false, I in turn spoke to the woman and agreed to discuss this matter with Dr. D.

When I mentioned to Dr. D. that Sandy claimed he told her there is no such thing as a Jarisch-Herxheimer reaction, he looked shocked. His version of the interaction went as follows:

> When Sandy told me she had a Jarisch-Herxheimer reaction I asked her to describe what happened after she started

the medication. She told me that her symptoms improved and stayed better for several months after she completed the medication. I explained to her that she could not have had a Jarisch-Herxheimer reaction since she would have felt worse instead of better, if she had indeed had one.

I was under the impression that she understood what I told her. Since I don't consider myself an expert on Lyme disease, I offered to refer her to an infectious disease specialist and she and her husband, who had accompanied her, seemed satisfied with the encounter when they left the office.

These kinds of misunderstandings probably occur more often than either doctors or patients realize. Perhaps before the encounter, the woman had misunderstood the meaning of a Jarisch-Herxheimer reaction to be a return or worsening of symptoms following treatment rather than a temporary worsening of symptoms during treatment. Therefore, when she relapsed months later and Dr. D. told her that she couldn't have had one, she misinterpreted him to mean there was no such thing. Perhaps it would have helped if Dr. D. had asked Sandy to repeat in her own words what he had explained to her to make sure it was clear.

Doctors use language that is offensive to patients

Several years into my illness, I was referred to the Mayo Clinic. I wanted to bring along as many of my previous medical records as possible, and since the visit was scheduled with relatively short notice, there wasn't time to mail records from our family clinic. Instead, I picked them up at the office and, although they were sealed, my curiosity prompted me to open them and read through them. I don't recall ever being quite so angry as I was at the time. It was clear that very little of what I had reported had been taken seriously. There were many inconsistencies between the information that I had reported and what was entered by the doctor. For instance, I clearly recalled a time the doctor had noted some pleurisy while listening to my chest. He questioned whether I'd had a recent cold. I told him I had not. He responded, "You must have." I again told him that I had no cough, no sniffles, no other signs of a cold. Yet, in my records he wrote, "Patient has pleurisy due to a recent cold."

The records were also riddled with phrases that seemed to undermine the validity of everything I had told him—phrases like "the patient denies" or "the patient claims." The wording seemed to confirm my earlier suspicions about the way my reports were received by doctors throughout most of my experience. I felt I was more or less on trial—and was guilty until proven innocent—guilty of feigning or imagining my symptoms until tests or exams could prove otherwise.

I realize now that I need not have taken it personally; it wasn't me—it is just the way doctors are trained to view patients and record information about them. It is part of the jargon that has precise meaning for doctors and doesn't necessarily have judgmental intent. But neither does it recognize patients' feelings.

Long after I reviewed my own records, Mary Hager, health reporter for *Newsweek* magazine, sent me an article by Laurie Fenlason, University of Michigan sociologist, about a study on the way doctors talk about patients. Fenlason describes the tendency of doctors to present their own observations as factual statements while casting patients' self-reported information in the realm of subjectivity stating that this is "among doctors' most insidious speech conventions." She confirms that, according to doctors' reports, patients invariably "admit," "claim," or "deny" while physicians "note" and "observe." An example she gave: "The patient states that she has been having uterine contractions every three minutes. She denies any rupture of the membrane."

Assuming that what the doctor says is fact, while the patient's report is constantly in question, she says, creates an unfair balance in the communication. "Studies of the doctor-patient relationship uniformly describe an asymmetry of knowledge and authority that allows doctors to promulgate a biomedical model of disease and to simultaneously undermine patients' own experience and understanding." She goes on to say, "Doctors who are learning the language of case presentations are going to be compelled subtly to adopt faith in the unquestioned knowledge of scientific information and to minimize the importance of the patient's history and subjective experience."

While from an intellectual perspective I can understand the reasons that doctors must be cautious about accepting as fact what is being reported by the patient, the emotional side of me cries that it isn't fair or appropriate not to give patients any credit for understanding their own bodies and for assessing when something is amiss.

Clearly, problems abound when too little credibility is given to the patients' observations, and when doctors rely entirely on objective evidence, since so much is missed on exams and tests. Fenlason concludes, "It's in our conversations that power relationships are established as much as in social institutions." Their language, she believes, reinforces their sense of power over the patient.

Perhaps it isn't feasible to change the language, and perhaps it is appropriate to always leave the door open for the possibility of faulty patient reports. Yet, if doctors are aware of the effect this language might have, perhaps they will be less likely to let it control the way they view and treat the patient and they will be able to keep a better balance, carefully listening to the patient instead of relying too heavily on their own observations and technical feedback. At the same time, patients need to realize that the physician's job is to see how the patient's subjective symptoms fit with clinical observations and test results based on knowledge of possible disease processes.

Patients don't understand a physician's reluctance to make a diagnosis

Doctors admit they are often reluctant to label a patient as having a serious illness until they are very certain since they are aware of possible repercussions. It could become more difficult for the patient to get a job, obtain health or life insurance, or change insurance companies once their disease has been confirmed. Doctors also feel it can be harmful to tell patients they have a potentially debilitating or life-threatening disease when there is a chance it could turn out to be something less ominous. When the reasons for being cautious about making a diagnosis are not explained to the patient, he might become angry and frustrated, believing the doctor is holding back information. I recall being told a number of times by physicians that I was better off without a diagnosis, which didn't make sense at the time because none of them explained their rationale for making this statement.

Medical jargon that is confusing to patients

I was surprised when the person assigned to the final editing of our patient self-help book, *When You're Sick and Don't Know Why*, commented that the vocabulary throughout seemed a bit sophisticated for a book geared for the general public. At the time she had not received the chapter written by John, so she was basing her conclusions on my writing, not on his as a physician. I did not and still do not have what I would consider to be an advanced technical vocabulary. However, apparently because I had spent a considerable amount of time poring through medical reports and medical books and talking with professionals, I had acquired a somewhat above average repertoire of medical jargon.

I suppose it becomes hard to recognize after awhile what is technical jargon and what is ordinary language once one has become accustomed to hearing and using the terminology peculiar to a given culture. I thought my book was written in pretty plain language. But what is clear depends on a person's previous exposure. It is no wonder that eight or more years of cramming medical jargon is likely to hinder a doctor's ability to communicate on the level of a lay person who perhaps has had no background in medical science. A doctor might think he is explaining clearly just what a patient has and what should be done about it when the patient is actually confused.

Adding to the problem of doctors speaking in a language that is "foreign" to many, people are usually nervous about being in the doctor's office. It is not surprising that patients often admit they understand or recall little of what the doctor said once they walk out the door. One study showed that patients, on average, recall only about 50 percent of what doctors tell them, leading to misuse of medication and slowed recovery.[3]

John tries to reduce these communication problems by making it a habit to ask his patients at the end of their visit two questions: "Is my explanation clear?" and "Do you have any additional questions?" Dr. Yarnall goes a step further by sending each patient a summary of what transpired during every visit and encouraging them to call if anything is not clear. While some doctors might groan over the additional time and paperwork, Yarnall says he finds it helpful to have staff members involved in the patient interview, so they can be involved in the communication. Nurse practitioners are becoming increasingly important figures in medical care, taking a more active role in many clinics by assuming some of the routine and time-consuming tasks in order to free doctors to handle more critical aspects of care.

9

SORTING OUT THE PHYSICAL AND PSYCHOLOGICAL COMPONENTS OF ILLNESS

A SIGNIFICANT obstacle to effectively managing illness in our society is the belief that everything must be organized into well-defined groups and be given a name. Our high need to categorize and label tends to lead us to deny the reality of anything we cannot put a name on. When it comes to illness, I believe this often hinders doctors' ability to help their patients. It also hinders the patients' ability to live as well as possible in spite of whatever ailments they are burdened with.

The desire to put labels on everything leads us to divide illnesses into two main categories—the psychogenic and the organic (physical). As a result, many doctors are quick to throw the problems of those who don't have clearly defined physical ailments into the psychological wastebasket, and patients who have undiagnosed symptoms easily become focused on proving they are "really sick," rather than on managing symptoms.

One of the greatest dilemmas faced by those in the medical profession is deciding how to best help the patient who is suffering from an illness that is not clearly defined. I have mulled over this chapter a great deal trying to decide how to best present the information I have gathered and the conclusions I have drawn. I finally decided to talk about what I believe are four key facts concerning the mind-body relationship, facts which have been confirmed by a number of doctors, psychologists and psychiatrists with whom I have discussed this over the years.

Fact 1. It is impossible to separate the mind from the body.

Rosalind M. Mance, psychiatrist at Emory University in Atlanta, Georgia, points out, "Science is just barely beginning to understand the intricate balance between the mind and the body"—and, I might add, the spirit. If one part is "diseased," every part will be affected. Diseases that disrupt the body's hormonal or chemical balance can present themselves as psychiatric disorders, and psychiatric disorders can be accompanied by very real physical symptoms.

Perhaps I can identify with this mind-body congruency more acutely than some. During this particular time of my life I feel quite well mentally, physically, and spiritually, for which I am grateful. However, in the past I have experienced significant depression and have also experienced a long-term illness that was eventually determined to have a physical cause.

As a young teenager, I struggled with depression—feelings of hopelessness, worthlessness and fear were almost daily companions. My depression was also accompanied by some physical ailments. My stomach was so "tied in knots" every morning before I went to school that I found it impossible to eat breakfast. When confronted with a situation in which I had to speak to someone other than my closest friends or family members, my heart would beat rapidly and my palms would sweat. I frequently suffered from insomnia and headaches. I even came down with infectious diseases such as colds and flu more often than my sister who was a bit feistier than I back then.

As I entered adulthood, on the surface I appeared to be coping with life fairly well, and usually I even felt considerably better than I had during my younger days. But smoldering beneath the surface were many of the same insecurities that had contributed to my earlier depression. These insecurities drove me to become a "people-pleaser" and a workaholic. Eventually the depression and anxiety began to push their way back to the surface. In response, I drove myself harder—the less time I had to "think," the easier I could suppress the depression. In order to boost my self-esteem, I worked even more diligently to do what I thought would make everybody else in my life happy and make me look good.

One day, when I was in my early thirties, I broke down. It started with uncontrollable crying jags. I consulted our family doctor thinking my hormones must be out of balance (which they probably were since the body reacts physically to stress). The doctor referred me to a psychiatrist, and a short time later I was hospitalized for twelve days with the diagnosis of "moderate clinical depression." That breakdown was a turning point in my life. Through much introspection and prayer, I learned a great deal about myself, gaining insights that set me on the path toward emotional and spiritual healing.

In 1981, three years after my brief hospitalization for

clinical depression, I woke up on a July morning feeling disoriented and weak. Within a matter of days I was plagued with a multitude of symptoms including all-over body pain that was concentrated in my joints, extreme weak spells, a constant urge to void, chest pain, chills and facial numbness. That summer turned out to be the beginning of over six years of contending with a fluctuating, sometimes bizarre array of symptoms, and a great many doctor visits and medical tests. Since early tests revealed no physical cause, my family doctor concluded I had "too many symptoms" and that it was "time to call a psychiatrist."

At the time of my mental breakdown three years earlier, I had not balked at his recommendation that I see a psychiatrist, but this time I protested. It just didn't make sense. I had not been depressed. I was not feeling out of control mentally. I just felt very ill. I knew in my heart that I was physically ill, not mentally. I spent the next several years feeling that I had to somehow prove it—in order to get a diagnosis and thus get help. During my struggle with this illness, I developed some attitudes and behaviors that are typical of hypochondriacs: I became focused on my symptoms, and I spent a lot of time in doctors' offices. I also dealt with a certain amount of depression and anxiety *because* of the uncertainty, pain and the forced changes in lifestyle and relationships resulting from my illness.

Eventually I developed what I believe was a healthy acceptance of my predicament, and through it all I learned to believe in myself. Today, as painful as the experience was, I am not sorry that it happened.

The point of sharing this brief synopsis is to illustrate that I have experienced first-hand how mental illness can affect the body and vice-versa. Yet, I believe there were some significant differences in the nature of the primarily physical illness and that of the primarily psychogenic illness. I hadn't been feeling anxious or out of control before my symptoms started in 1981. Things had been going relatively well in my life. Also, I didn't lack the mental energy that I did during the 1979 depression, nor did I feel there was anything that I needed to escape from. I had the desire to carry on as I had before the illness; I was simply too sick to do so. And no matter how hard I tried to convince myself my symptoms were a figment of my imagination or force myself to function normally, I couldn't.

While many people with ongoing undiagnosed symptoms are told they are depressed, the conclusions of Dr. Paul Cheney, a Lake Tahoe physician who is interested in chronic fatigue syndrome, make a great deal of sense to me. He says:

> Depression requires a loss of interest in everything. These [chronic fatigue] patients are just the opposite. They're terribly concerned about what their symptoms mean. They can't function. They can't work. Many are petrified. But they do not lack interest in their surroundings. [1]

Nor did I while I was sick, nor do the people I continue to hear from on a daily basis who desperately want to know what is wrong with them and do not believe they are depressed.

Fact 2. It is very difficult to discern to what degree an illness is attributable to a mind dysfunction and to what degree a body dysfunction.

The answer to whether an illness is more physical or more mental lies within the patient. Although suggestions might be made by a doctor, except in extreme cases the patient is the one who must decide to accept psychological evaluation and treatment if it is to be effective.

Many doctors base their diagnoses on inability to find evidence of a physical problem, but this doesn't make sense in light of the number of illnesses that often do not present any "concrete" physical findings, or that have physical changes that doctors are missing. I met one woman who had a nine-pound abdominal tumor surgically removed after being told for nearly a year by several doctors, including a psychiatrist, that her abdominal pain was emotionally based. When the pain became so bad that she walked doubled over, the true culprit was discovered; by then she was told the noncancerous tumor was so invasive that she might not live through the surgery. Fortunately, she came through it very well.

Another woman, Brenda Selberg, suffered excruciating pain and nausea from a chronically infected appendix for three years before doctors discovered the problem. There were times that for months on end practically all she did was lay in bed and cry. The reality of her pain was discounted by doctors and, subsequently, by her family and friends. A laparoscopy finally indicated a mass in her lower right abdomen and surgery revealed that her colon had wrapped itself around her appendix, keeping it from rupturing, while the appendix had slowly leaked poison into her system. Brenda's bladder had also become adhered to the surrounding scar tissue from the repeated infections. Brenda recalls that the three doctors involved in her care—a gynecologist, a surgeon and her family doctor—were incredulous that she had been able to endure such severe pain for so long. So much for doctors' ability to assess the reality or degree of someone's pain before they know the cause.

I consider Rosalind Mance's insights into mind-body components of illness especially valuable for a number of reasons. Although she currently practices psychiatry, before going into that branch of medicine she completed a residency in general internal medicine and practiced in that realm for a few years. Therefore, I suspect that she has more insight than someone who has been trained extensively in just one of these areas. Even though psychiatrists are medical doctors, she says that they often don't "feel" like medical doctors because they have very little hands-on experience in diagnosing and treating the physical components of illness.

The depth of Dr. Mance's empathy for people with undiagnosed medical conditions and the associated emotional distress is, in mxy estimation, paralleled by only a few other medical professionals that I have met. When I questioned whether a personal experience had contributed to her interest in the emotional impact of illness, especially in difficult-to-diagnose illness, she shared the following story:

> I suppose that I can trace my interest in medicine in general, as well as my interest in the mind-body connection, back to my childhood. Until I was about seven years old, my mother suffered from an undiagnosed illness that involved marginally psychotic episodes followed by seizures. For years, doctors hinted that her problems were emotional. Eventually she was diagnosed as having hypoglycemia caused by a pancreatic tumor. It was very rare to have this sort of condition; hers was one of the first identified cases.
>
> Even after she was diagnosed she continued to suffer effects of the disease because she denied that anything was wrong until she started going into one of her episodes. My responsibility, when I was six, seven and eight years old, was to force her to drink sugared orange juice at the first sign of craziness.
>
> Eventually she had the tumor surgically removed and the symptoms abated. I was impressed by the fact that all of her acting out—her weirdness—was ultimately 100 percent due to a somatic [physical] lesion.

Physicians can usually link their decisions to go into medicine to things that happened in childhood—often they have experiences that instill in them a desire to "make things right." That's why they also often have a built-in resistance to acceptance of not always being able to put things right. The "if I can't find it, it doesn't exist" mentality comes out of that.

In my case, because of my earlier experiences with depression and the fact that tests showed no organic abnormalities, it was somewhat understandable that many doctors were convinced that my condition was psychogenic. However, I have heard countless stories from people who said they had no history of mental problems and were told at some point before being diagnosed with physical symptoms that their symptoms were "imaginary." Bonnie Harrison is just one example:

> I first realized that something was wrong in 1985. I consulted a dermatologist for a big, ugly rash on my back. While there, I also complained of extreme fatigue and weakness that had come on about the same time as the rash.
>
> The doctor dismissed the fatigue and weakness as "normal for a woman who works full-time and has a family to care for." He prescribed a variety of topical treatments and when they didn't help, he told me to lie in the sun. I convinced myself that he was right. I was probably just stressed out. I had never had a medical problem before and it didn't occur to me to question the doctor.
>
> Although I learned later that lying in the sun probably aggravated my problems rather than helping, I was determined to follow the doctor's advice. I struggled through the next two years. Every time I returned to the doctor he reaffirmed that I just had "a woman's problem."
>
> Finally, I got so bad I could hardly drag myself to work any more. One day I decided that I knew I wasn't crazy—

I was really sick. I didn't care if the doctor perceived my condition as a woman's problem. I knew there was more wrong, and I went back to the doctor and told him so.

Tests at the University of Minnesota showed severe impairment in the functioning of Bonnie's liver and kidneys, causing doctors to suspect lupus. Although initial blood work appeared normal, later more extensive blood work at Johns Hopkins confirmed the diagnosis of lupus.

Stories like Bonnie's are far from rare. The data in the accompanying table are taken from the same group of 232 patients discussed in earlier chapters.

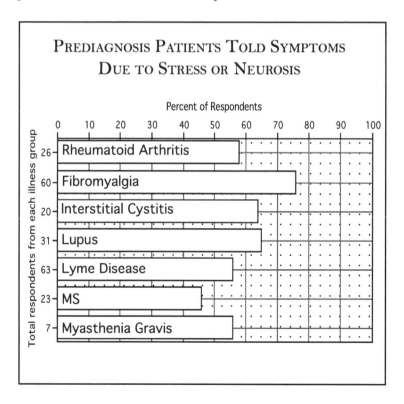

PREDIAGNOSIS PATIENTS TOLD SYMPTOMS DUE TO STRESS OR NEUROSIS

Over 50 percent of the people in six of the groups surveyed were told at some point that their symptoms were not "real" or were caused by stress. While broad generalizations can't be made from this relatively small group, the results tend to reinforce my belief that psychological mislabeling is an issue. According to Dr. Ezzo, it is not hard to find stress factors on which to blame people's illnesses:

> When I do yearly physicals, I ask patients about their stress levels. I find it interesting that only about two percent say they are not significantly stressed. Everyone has stress. If you are looking for a stress factor, you will find it in 98 percent of people's lives.

While some doctors agree there is a tendency to over-psychologize symptoms when a diagnosis is elusive, others remain convinced that a large portion of the patient population is suffering from "imaginary" symptoms. Many doctors are also convinced that the majority of people with less well-defined illnesses like chronic fatigue syndrome and fibromyalgia are most likely depressed and have no underlying organic disease. When I ask them why they believe this, their response invariably is that these people have no objective signs of illness—and they "can just tell" the patient is neurotic. There is really no scientific data, nor can there be, to support these judgments. I find it ironic that doctors are willing to base their conclusions on feelings, since in every other area of medicine they are very concerned with having scientific data to support their conclusions—everything else in medicine must be proved. When you look at the number of neurological and arthritic diseases that often take years to diagnose, and the number of people who claim they were labeled neurotic before being diagnosed with an organic disease, the evidence suggests that doctors are relatively poor at making judgments in these areas. Basing a psychogenic diagnosis on lack of evidence of a physical cause is rather presumptuous given the complexities of the diagnostic process and the fallibilities of medical testing.

Perhaps this in an issue about which some of my physician friends and I will always disagree. Yet, I share Dr. Mance's dream that "someday scientists will have an even better understanding of the mind-body connection." She says:

> My fantasy is that in the next 50 years we will have a much better understanding of the neuropsychology of the whole group of disorders like fibromyalgia and chronic fatigue syndrome. Perhaps we will learn they do involve the brain in some way. We just can't separate the mind from the rest of the body.
>
> Although doctors often assume that if antidepressants help a patient's condition it is psychogenic, that isn't necessarily true. Antidepressants are used for a wide range of disorders, not just depressive disorders.
>
> We are making new discoveries all the time. Tricyclic antidepressants are emerging as useful agents in neuropathic pain control. There is a general lack of understanding among physicians about where we are with these drugs.

As I interviewed physicians I found that, in general, the women gave more credence to fibromyalgia and chronic fatigue syndrome than did their male colleagues. Cate McKegney admits there are still many unknowns when it comes to these illnesses and that current treatments are "shotgun" and diagnoses don't address the etiology. Yet she says, "A diagnosis is the way into a support group these days, and support groups are one avenue of helping these people cope."

Fact 3. Having an ongoing unnamed illness can make you a little crazy.

Dr. Mance brings up an important point about people with chronic undiagnosed illness:

> Whatever personality a person has going into a chronic undiagnosed illness, their coping mechanisms are broken down by the experience of living with the ongoing pain and the uncertainty. The personality changes along with the body.

She reinforces my belief that people with undiagnosed illness often become rather neurotic—even people who were quite emotionally stable beforehand. Dealing for months or years with life-disrupting symptoms for which there is no explanation and little compassion is a "soul-sized battle" according to the authors of *Sick and Tired of Feeling Sick and Tired*. I should emphasize the term "life-disrupting." Most people can deal with some degree of pain and uncertainty. I experienced symptoms of carpal tunnel syndrome that disrupted my sleep for about ten years before being properly diagnosed. When my family doctor didn't have an explanation for the numbness in my hands and pain in my arm early on, I didn't make it a life pursuit to find the cause. The illness that came on in 1981 was different—it was much more frightening and much more disruptive—it refused to let me brush it aside.

While some people with undiagnosed symptoms might become obsessive about them and talk about them too much, others might seem inappropriately serene or cheerful about them. Both of these behaviors are commonly cited in psychogenic illnesses as well. Recalling the circumstances surrounding the addition of involuntary choreaform movements to my own repertoire of symptoms and the reaction of the first neurologist who observed me, I realize now that my response probably seemed inappropriate to him. Even though the movement was bizarre, both my husband and I had by then grown accustomed to strange occurrences. (My other symptoms then included numbness, collapsing from weakness, uncoordinated gait and loss of bladder control.) By then, we were both exhausted emotionally and unsure any more how to respond to this even stranger new symptom. We were also probably into some denial. Therefore, at the time I saw the doctor, I was matter-of-fact about the jerking. In another context, I know I would have been alarmed by it, and my husband would have taken me right to an emergency room.

People with ongoing undiagnosed symptoms are often placed in a paradoxical situation, being encouraged to deny the reality of their symptoms when getting past the denial is recognized as the first step in managing the grief associated with any loss. And there can be many losses associated with an ongoing illness: Loss of a sense of well-being, loss of employment, loss of ability to participate in familiar pastimes and hobbies, loss of social life, and loss of a sense of control.

Even when physicians don't question a patient's mental stability, the patient often questions it himself. "The worst thing for many with undiagnosed illness is the self-torment," says Dr. Mance. "There is the notion that if it doesn't have a name—if they can't understand it, they must be making it up. They often agonize over whether they are just trying to get out of something or be more disabled than they really are. They ask themselves over and over, Am I crazy?"

Even though most people with undiagnosed illnesses do question their own sanity, they might adamantly deny that possibility to doctors, since there is usually a stronger intuition telling them they are dealing with a physical illness, and they fear the doctor will stop looking for the cause. If they are reassured that their doctor won't close the door to exploring physical possibilities, they are much more likely to admit their own doubts and to explore psychological issues as well. I recently interviewed Lianne Anderson, a woman who was diagnosed with myasthenia gravis nearly ten years ago. Before the diagnosis, when her doctor told her he believed her symptoms were emotionally based, she responded, "I'm willing to consider the possibility that this is a psychological problem if you are willing to consider that it might be physical."

Few physicians realize the torment people go through when they are being told or are trying to convince themselves they should be able to function normally, but they can't. I constantly struggled with guilt, wondering if I was really putting my family and friends through worry and spending hard-earned money on doctor bills for nothing. I wasn't at peace until I was finally able to stop questioning my mental stability, accept my unnamed illness and start learning to live the best I could with my symptoms.

As I talked with doctors I found that some were very torn about the best way to handle undiagnosed patients who they suspect are suffering from psychogenic symptoms. There is a real fear among them of confirming what might be delusional illnesses. One doctor explained that he had been working with a woman who was diagnosed with fibromyalgia by another doctor. A number of unsuccessful remedies were tried for her pain. He finally referred her for acupuncture, which she reported was helping. Yet, rather than being happy that he had been able to help her, he was distraught because he believed he was really only helping her to avoid confronting underlying emotional problems. "But I know her illness isn't real," he lamented.

I explained to this physician that, in my view, even if underlying psychological problems were the primary cause of the woman's symptoms, he had done the right thing. He was more likely to gain her trust by helping her find ways to manage the physical pain. Had he discounted her symptoms and refused to offer help, he probably would have contributed to her distress, and perhaps sent her scurrying to a different doctor. By agreeing to work with her, he will probably get to know her better over time, and perhaps eventually he will find opportunities to tactfully broach psychological issues as well. On the other hand, new evidence might eventually prove that her symptoms are physically based.

Having talked to thousands of patients and family members of patients, I am convinced that doctors do harm more often by refusing to validate symptoms than they do by validating them. Rosalind Mance reinforced how difficult it can be to assess someone else's pain and the mysteries of the pain experience:

> When my two children were younger they were both constantly getting ear infections. Each time my daughter got one, she was obviously in pain from the onset and, therefore, was always treated early. My son, on the other hand, never complained of pain until his ear drum was literally bulging from the pressure. I would then take him to a doctor who would exclaim, "My goodness, how long has this been going on!"

Indeed, there is much to be learned in regard to the whys and hows of the way people experience pain.

It is possible for a doctor to leave the door open to exploring psychological factors, yet at the same time validate the patient's symptoms and reassure him that he won't be abandoned. In Chapter 3, we discussed some of the things that doctors can say to help ease people through the prediagnosis period.

John confirms that many of his patients are open to talking to a psychologist when he explains that a psychological evaluation will just provide one more piece of information:

> If patients feel like they are being dumped off, they are not likely to agree to see a psychologist. But if they are reassured that we will keep working together on finding an answer, they are usually pretty open to doing so. In fact, once they go, many of them actually find it helpful to have someone who is willing to listen and to help them deal with the difficult issue of having an illness with no name. It is also helpful for patients who are dealing with newly diagnosed chronic illnesses.

When counseling undiagnosed patients, Dr. Mance explains the importance of just being with that person in the experience:

> Validating their experience, touching them in some way is part of the healing. Only when you can be with the patient in the place they are, can you work together on ways to sort out the etiological factors—only then can you start looking at options that will either help the patient move out of the illness or learn ways to manage it.
>
> It is a lot of work dealing with people who have chronic undiagnosed illness and it's important to have a quality support network to help find effective solutions. I keep close ties with pain clinics and with caring doctors in a variety of specialties. But I still see myself as the primary support.

According to Dr. Mance, the way physicians respond to difficult-to-diagnose patients depends very much on the way they are taught and how open they are to looking at their own role in helping people. She says:

In the past, doctors were there to support people through the natural course of disease. Today, physicians are taught in medical school to cure. Yet, there are very few physical ailments we can actually cure. Medical education plays a critical role in developing supportive physicians who accept patients' perceptions of their experience as key to finding the right therapy.

Fact 4. People often find it easier being told they have a serious disease than dealing with an undiagnosed illness.

Doctors often find it difficult to understand why a patient would rather receive word of a serious medical condition than be sick and not know why. In fact, now that I have been well for over six years, I find it difficult to put myself in the position of wishing I could have a diagnosis even if it meant I had a crippling disease.

I recall the first time I spoke at an MS support group after I was diagnosed, treated, and once again a physically healthy person. As I studied people in the room, some of them in wheelchairs, some with speech impediments and hand tremors, I found it hard to believe that I would have been happy, at one point in my life, to be told I had MS. It wasn't that I wanted to have MS or that I wanted to be sick. I just was sick, and the symptoms had been going on long enough that I was convinced I had something serious that wasn't likely to just go away. The symptoms were significantly impacting my life. A diagnosis would have given me something to rest on, perhaps some degree of certainty to begin structuring my life around.

Dr. Savett confirms that people generally deal with the bad news of serious illness very well. After some initial mourning, he says, people often find their lives richer for the experience of becoming aware of their mortality. "The uncertainty of not knowing is much more difficult for people to deal with," he adds.

People are sometimes defensive about psychogenic suggestions, which I have learned only causes doctors to become more suspicious that the illness is a psychiatric problem. In *When You're Sick and Don't Know Why*, I attempted to clarify why psychogenic diagnoses are often resented, even feared by patients. Here is a summary of the complex assortment of emotions that are often triggered by psychiatric explanations for physical symptoms.[3] They include:

Disbelief: People have often already questioned the reality of their symptoms before consulting a doctor and have determined in their minds that the symptoms are not psychogenic.

Increased anxiety: *My doctor isn't taking me seriously and is going to stop trying to find the cause. What am I going to do now?*

Anger: *The doctor isn't giving me credit for knowing when something is wrong with my own body.*

Humiliation: *What are people going to think if I tell them my doctor believes this is all in my head? Will my family and friends think I am just lazy or looking for attention?*

Dismay: The idea of being labeled a hypochondriac is not a great alternative. A doctor's affirmation or lack of affirmation of a physical condition can make a significant impact on the way others respond to a person. How many employers would tolerate an employee who offers hypochondriasis as an excuse for poor work performance or attendance? A physical diagnosis is much more likely to draw understanding and a willingness to compromise. I work with a woman who has had to adjust her work schedule to accommodate caring for her ailing son. Her manager has been very understanding, allowing her to work fewer, more flexible hours. I wonder how that same manager would respond if the woman announced that she could not work on schedule because she was neurotic.

Realizing my interest in the issue, a neighbor shared that she worked with a woman who was continually complaining of pain in her arm. Since doctors couldn't find anything wrong, everyone in the office was convinced the woman was a hypochondriac, and no one offered sympathy. They felt guilty when it was eventually learned that the woman's pain was cause by a fatal cancer. All of us need to be careful not to pass judgment about the validity of someone else's pain.

Self-doubt: Until they have a diagnosis, people tend to question whether they are imagining or exaggerating their symptoms. When doctors suggest they are, it adds to their confusion. Trying to sort it all out, the patient often becomes more focused on symptoms, becomes more tense and the symptoms are likely to feel worse.

Many doctors admit there can be frustration in dealing with patients who have vague symptoms like fatigue and weakness but whose tests are normal. Dr. Savett offered some helpful insights drawn from his 30 years of working with patients:

> I find it very easy to talk to patients in these situations. When I suspect that stress or depression are contributing to their illnesses, I ask them to share what is going on in their lives. They are usually very open. Rather than telling them their symptoms are "all in your head," I ask them,

"To what extent do you think other factors in your life are affecting the way you feel?" They either respond, "I do have a lot on my mind, it probably is affecting how I feel," or they might say, "I know I have a lot on my mind, but I don't think it is related to my symptoms.

Or I might suggest that a person's symptoms are related to stress or depression and then ask, "Does that sound reasonable to you?" Turning it around and asking for their opinion validates the experience. People know if they are depressed or not.

Like John, Dr. Savett proves that it is possible to broach psychological possibilities without alienating the patient if the subject is handled in a sensitive, open-minded manner.

According to Dr. Ezzo, because many patients have a "hands-off" attitude when it comes to including depression in the differential diagnosis, she also has found it important to be careful about her approach:

> I still have to come through the back door to get patients interested in exploring depression as a possibility when they come in with classic symptoms—early morning wakening, psychomotor slowing, difficulty concentrating. However, when I am honest, explaining my personal belief that depression is biochemically based, they are more receptive and are willing to try medication to see if it will improve their sleep patterns and thus help the symptoms.

A major fear of patients who are confronted with a possible psychological diagnosis is that they are going to have to deal with it on their own, says Cate McKegney:

> Part of my role as a family doctor is to reassure patients that I will not abandon them in either regard, since as a family practitioner both psychological and physical illnesses are in my arena.

For a long time I was regularly seeing a patient who had an undiagnosed illness. The only thing I did was listen to her and tell her that I wasn't abandoning her. I hadn't a clue as to what was going on. We had done the right tests, but the tests we had at the time were just not good enough. Eventually we were able to diagnose her with hepatitis C, a disease that has not been well known until more sensitive tests were developed just recently. Because I and other doctors involved in her case had taken good histories, when the test became available we thought to test her for it.

The mind-body issue is enormously complex. When it comes to differentiating the truly physical from the truly psychogenic, the uncertainties of medical science are glaring and in this regard the doctor-patient relationship is truly tested. In an article printed in the *Journal of the American Medical Association*, authors N. P. Wray and J. A. Friedland say the false assumption of psychological illness based on nothing more than uncertainty, insecurity and ignorance is "probably the most common error made in medicine. On the other hand the physical illnesses of psychiatric patients go underdiagnosed or undiagnosed." [*]

I would be negligent if I didn't include in this chapter some discussion of truly psychogenic illnesses since their existence is undeniable. Hypochondriasis, conversion reaction disorders and other psychiatric illnesses can deceive the afflicted into believing they are suffering from physical ailments when their bodies are quite healthy. There are also people who feign or exaggerate illnesses or injuries to get out of work or for monetary gain. "It can be tricky to discern when these factors are part of an illness," confirms Dr. Ezzo. However, she adds, "In these cases there are often inconsistencies in the patient's stories and they seem intent on playing up their 'disabilities.'"

There are also differences in people's perceptions of their conditions, Ezzo says:

> I am often intrigued by what I see as a subgroup of people who are so afraid of pain that they don't realize you can have pain and yet continue to be functional. There are times when patients want me to confirm they are disabled and I can't agree. These people usually don't return.

Dr. Brian Fallon, assistant professor of clinical psychiatry and director of the somatic disorders program at Columbia University, works with many patients who have physical ailments that are difficult to diagnose or treat. He also works with those who suffer from true psychogenic illnesses such as hypochondriasis. Hypochondriacs, he says, come in two varieties: those who recognize the irrationality of their fears about illness and those who are almost completely delusional.

> Patients exhibit varying degrees of insight. Some have a good deal of insight into the irrationality of their fears, others have no insight at all, and some have wavering insight. Those with wavering insight might readily admit their illness fears are unfounded some days, but on days when they are experiencing symptoms, they might be again convinced they are seriously ill.
>
> Patients with a high degree of insight are likely to consult a psychiatrist for help, while those who are completely delusional do not like coming to see a psychiatrist and rarely do so unless they are dragged in by family members.

Fallon goes on to explain that at times it is hard to tell whether one is dealing with hypochondriasis or a difficult-to-diagnose physical problem:

> You have to make sure you listen to the patient, do every appropriate test, and consider the possibility of unusual dis-

eases. You also have to take into consideration the character of the patient. There are people who hate feeling sick and whose goal is to be well again and get back to living as normal a life as possible. There are others who readily take on the sick role, dwelling on their symptoms and becoming very dependent on the support of others. In the latter case, when all physical possibilities are ruled out, you are led in the direction of a primarily psychological diagnosis.

When diagnosing somatoform disorders we also look back at the patient's early history. If their complaints have existed since childhood or adolescence, we are more likely to diagnose a somatoform disorder [a disorder for which there is no physical explanation for the symptoms—also called psychogenic or somatization disorder].

Fallon admits that, in reality, it is impossible to ever completely rule out physical disorders given the imperfections and inconsistencies of medical testing. It is also important to keep in mind that somatoform disorders cannot be controlled "at will" by the patient; brain chemistry changes are also involved. And Fallon believes that people with such illnesses do experience physical symptoms much more acutely than others do. He points out that many people who are suffering from obsessional illnesses respond well to medication; in a pilot study on the use of Prozac, 70 percent of those who had been diagnosed as hypochondriacal improved while taking the drug.

According to Fallon, people sometimes experience physical symptoms as a result of trauma or unresolved grief:

> I've met patients who were irrationally terrified about their physical symptoms. In some of these cases, when we explored their history, we discovered they had recently suffered a major loss, perhaps the death of a close relative. Their grief then became internalized, manifesting itself as

a physical symptom. Once these people start working through their grief and identifying their repressed emotions, they get well. Sometimes it only takes a few months of therapy.

Fallon does not classify fibromyalgia and chronic fatigue syndrome along with somatoform illnesses as do some in his profession:

> There have been some articles published in psychiatric journals claiming these syndromes are modern forms of abnormal behavior similar to neurasthenia in the early 1900s. I don't think this is true in many cases. There is growing evidence to indicate the presence of immunological problems in these patients. Chronic fatigue syndrome, for example, may represent the last common denominator for various infectious diseases like Epstein Barr virus and Lyme disease. An infection, bacterial or viral, may have triggered the immune system to start fighting not only the invading organism but also parts of one's own body. The chemicals released by the abnormally activated immune system may then cause symptoms of chronic fatigue syndrome.

Fallon admits there is a shortage of medical doctors who are trained to deal tactfully with people who are suspected of having psychogenic illnesses. He adds:

> The health care model has traditionally been over-oriented toward "cure" rather than "care." Thus when physicians can't make the diagnosis or provide a cure, instead of admitting their own inabilities, they project their unhappiness and frustration on the patient by saying in effect, "You're a crock, go see a psychiatrist." I think that will change along with changes in our health care system. We are moving toward a more family practice centered health care model. Family practitioners receive a fair amount of training in psychiatry. I

currently work out of a family practice clinic. Some patients I would normally see are being treated very well by family medicine doctors. These physicians have a sophisticated whole-person approach. They are particularly skilled at working with patients whose diagnosis is uncertain and with those who have chronic medical problems that can't be cured with modern medicine. Through empathic listening and judicious medical interventions, these physicians can help patients maximize their potential despite the physical limitations imposed by illness.

10

THE MAKING OF A GOOD DOCTOR

After each [doctor] visit, I feel at peace, and that's half the battle. [1]

—Ann L. Drake

I FREQUENTLY receive unsolicited feedback about physicians who practice in the towns and cities near my home. One particular rheumatologist has been hailed as a great man by a few of his patients and a real bungler by others. Since personalities are diverse and people's needs and experiences vary greatly, there are bound to be differences in the way people perceive individual doctors. However, some physicians almost invariably receive high praise from their patients, and others are frequently complained about, says Dr. John Butler, who is responsible for performance reviews of colleagues. He adds, "Some doctors are very frustrated. They don't have the tools or the experience needed to develop a good rapport with their patients."

It goes without saying that a good doctor needs to be well educated about the human body in health and disease, skilled in procedures he is required to perform, and up to date on new information. However, much of what is learned in medical school is inapplicable or forgotten. One doctor admitted, "I estimate that 60 percent of what was taught in medical school classrooms I never used, 30 percent was incorrect and about 10 percent was potentially valuable." [2] Clearly, an "A" medical student does not necessarily translate to a good doctor.

And since medical science is changing at a dizzying speed, keeping pace with the new discoveries in medicine is virtually impossible for physicians. In spite of considerable time spent reading medical journals and attending continuing education courses, many of them say they feel inadequate when it comes to staying current with new information.

Most people agree that being a good doctor goes beyond education and technology, but opinions differ more when it comes to defining just what constitutes a good doctor. My own concept of a good doctor comes from years of interviews and considerable personal experience. The doctors I have encountered include family practitioners and a variety of specialists including neurologists, urologists, infectious disease specialists, psychiatrists, rheumatologists and internists. All but a few of them, I believe, were acceptably competent in their fields. I sensed that most were trying their best to help me and I would not consider them "bad" doctors.

But the field of medicine calls for excellence. A good doctor must strive to transcend the knowledge and the technical skills. Only the doctor who takes appropriate advantage of the enormous healing power inherent to the role can be a top-notch physician. A doctor who learns how to establish a rapport that promotes healing, whether or not an actual cure is close at hand, will be most effective in helping patients move closer to wellness.

Of the more than two dozen doctors I encountered during my illness between 1981 and 1987, a few were truly exceptional. One woman called after reading my first book to thank me for writing about this "great" man, referring to John Witek. Her husband has MS and is one of John's patients. "You have no idea how much easier it has been for us to deal with this illness with Dr. Witek's support," she said. Many others have contacted me since then saying they have found their "own Dr. Witek." Despite living with difficult illnesses, they say the support of a good doctor has made their lives so much better, enabling them to live well in spite of their illnesses. The qualities they describe as helpful do not include intelligence or technical ability. Rather they center on respectful, nonjudgmental and compassionate care.

I noted that doctors who are particularly good with their patients are constantly contemplating ways to improve communication. Dr. Savett says, "The doctor-patient relationship is precious to the healing process. When an encounter with a patient doesn't go well, I always sit down afterward and analyze the situation, try to determine why. Without naming the patient, I often discuss the situation with my wife, who is a medical social worker, to get her insight. In the process I am often able to find ways to resolve the problem and develop a better rapport."

Dr. Savett describes "difficult" patients as generally falling into one of three categories: those who have illnesses which are difficult to diagnose, those who have a diagnosis but are not responding as well as expected to treatment, and those with whom rapport is difficult to establish. He says that he has found it relatively easy to work with and to help people in all of these groups when he takes a little extra time to ask about the bigger picture. "I find it very easy to ask about what is happening in these people's lives. Often there are psychological or social issues which contribute to their illness or hinder the healing process and just acknowledging them opens the door to resolution."

Dr. Gregory Silvis says, "Healers have played a central role in every society, even without the impressive equipment and knowledge we have acquired in recent years. They must have had something that made them successful. Since they didn't have the technology, it must have had something to do with the words they used, with the relationships they formed. Imagine what would happen if we could capture the communication skills they had and combine them with what we have acquired. We'd have the most powerful healing system the world has ever seen."

I believe that some doctors today *have* captured the best of both worlds. They *have* learned to balance their knowledge and technical abilities with excellent people skills. These doctors have also reached a level of maturity in their practices that allows them to graciously admit their own limitations to themselves and to their patients. The way I see it, these doctors have a key trait that is essential to the making of a "good" doctor, and that trait is humility.

Humility translates to:

Honesty about personal limitations and the shortcomings of medicine in general. I discovered that most physicians with a reputation for having good rapport with their patients are not afraid to say "I don't know" and are willing to take time to discuss the uncertainties of medicine with their patients.

Willingness to consult with other doctors or refer a patient on when answers aren't clear. Sometimes a doctor is too close to a situation to see the obvious. A good doctor recognizes the value of a fresh perspective. John affirms that many a medical mystery is resolved by calling in a new doctor.

A maturity level that allows joy rather than jealousy when some-one else comes up with the right answer. Although John worked with me during the last two years of my illness, he was not the one who actually made the diagnosis or successfully treated my condition. Yet, he was obviously thrilled by the events. A doctor who cares more about the well-being of his patients than about attaining personal glory is a gift.

Good listening skills. Realizing the patient holds the key to making the diagnosis and finding the best treatment proto-col, a good doctor recognizes the importance of taking time to really listen to what the patient is saying.

Open-mindedness. When it comes to suggestions from col-leagues, patients and outside sources, a humble doctor is likely to keep an open mind rather than shutting out potentially helpful ideas. It is interesting that many remedies that were discounted or ignored by the medical profession previously are now becoming proven remedies. Grandma's chicken soup, for instance, has been scientifically shown to have healing properties.

A true sense of humility is the trait in a physician that is most likely to draw the greatest respect and degree of coop-eration from patients. In contrast, arrogance and the per-ception of arrogance cause animosity in the relationship and increase the likelihood that the doctor will miss opportuni-ties to help a patient.

It was refreshing to talk with many physicians who obvi-ously delight in their work. Here are some additional com-ments about their own practices and medical practice in gen-eral from doctors who have good reputations for working with patients.

On the physician's role:

You have to get away from the "find it and fix it" mode to a much broader role. I see my practice as more of an interfacing with the patient—as part of the process toward that person's healing—rather than the person doing the curing. I listen to the patient, filter the information and draw on the large body of knowledge to offer input.

—Robert Wagner

I give my patients a lot of control in their own therapy unless the situation is life-threatening. I consider myself their consultant. I explain the results of the exam and lab tests, discuss the pros and cons of treating or not treating and explain all the options. Then I let them make the decisions. It's their health. They should make the decisions.

—Mary Ezzo

On being friends with patients:

At one time it was thought best not be friends with our patients—we were advised not to get too close. I find the opposite true.

—Stephen Yarnall

When the doctor is willing to share a little of himself with the patient, it is a gesture of respect. It is like saying, "I trust you." When he doesn't, it is like saying, "I don't trust you, you are not worthy of being brought into my world; the only reason I'm relating to you at all is because it's my job."

However, there is a fairly delicate balance. You can be friends, but it has to be kept on a certain level. If the friendship moves too far outside the professional arena, it becomes difficult to deal with the medical problems in a balanced way. It becomes too easy to give in, and perhaps prescribe something the patient asks for that might not be good for him. And people might feel uncomfortable if the doctor talks too much about himself.

—Robert Wagner

Although I like to keep a certain professional level to the relationship, I share my personal life with my patients. Younger people, especially, relate better to situations when I can use my own life as an example. Getting to know the personal side of my patients' lives is half the healing.

—Mary Ezzo

On good doctors:

A good doctor is good at listening, good at explaining, good at comforting. Perhaps most important a good doctor knows what he is good at and is not too proud to make referrals when he knows that someone else might be better.

—John Butler

On honesty:

It's important not to keep secrets. I used to send a letter off to every patient after the office visit; now I dictate a progress note concerning the visits. The patient can read this and understand that I'm not keeping anything a secret.

—Stephen Yarnall

On spending enough time with patients:

Medicine can get to be hard work if a physician starts overbooking patients. It is important to regulate your schedule so you can spend enough time with each patient. Then the work becomes more satisfying—more like the old style of medicine.

—John Witek

I spend quality time, rather than quantity. I try to be efficient with time as well. I have a lot of people helping with mundane tasks and with history taking in each clinic session. I then have more time to discuss the personal side of the illness with the patient.

—Stephen Yarnall

I find that sitting down and meeting the needs of the patient takes less time than somehow shadowboxing my way out of the interview. The patient comes in with an agenda, and it's much better to address that agenda head on.

—Mary Ezzo

Acting rushed or hurried creates all kinds of negatives. If you can't act interested in what the patient is saying, you might as well cancel the visit. A reasonably competent physician should be able to manage the time issue.

—John Witek

On the patient interview:

The politics of medicine drive me crazy, but once I'm in the exam room one-on-one with the patient, it's very enjoyable. That's what is real.

—Mary Ezzo

We can be upset with insurance companies, forms and hospital meetings, but most of the physician's time is spent seeing patients. If that doesn't go well, everything else becomes pretty minor. A physician who doesn't enjoy interviewing patients is going to be a pretty frustrated person.

—John Witek

I start the interview with lighthearted chatting, often sharing a little of myself with the patient. I never tell a patient there is nothing we can do. I always say there is a lot we can do, that we'll work together on finding solutions. This sets the relationship on a positive note. When dealing with difficult patients, I try not to respond to anger with anger.

—Stephen Yarnall

You can be having a bad day, have someone in the hospital who is not doing well. But when you go in to see the next patient you must start with a clean slate. You have to go in reasonably prepared and upbeat. You can't bring in baggage from earlier visits or from the day before.

—John Witek

On getting too involved:

It's important to have a mixture of compassion and caring on one hand, and creative indifference on the other. My view is that no problem is major. I see the problems of this life as temporary. Therefore, the problems we encounter here are temporary, which helps me from becoming too distraught over the suffering of my patients.

—Stephen Yarnall

These doctors and many of the other doctors interviewed for this book confirmed that doctors and patients can enjoy rewarding relationships. If doctors want to take time to develop positive rapports with their patients, they can. And when they do, it can make an enormous difference in the satisfaction for both parties while greatly enhancing the healing potential of the relationship.

The doctor often sets the tone of the entire office. I noticed that even the atmosphere in the waiting room could impact the way I felt. If I was welcomed by warm, friendly receptionists, I immediately felt more relaxed about the visit. If they acted cold and unfriendly, I became more tense. I was particularly impressed to see doctors who met people in the lounge and personally escort them into the exam room.

In their own journals, colleagues are noting that because alternative healers usually have limited treatment options, they concentrate on the most important treatment option of all—the healer-patient relationship—and they ask, "Could alternative healers, despite their weaknesses, be in effect showing the medical profession the path to more effective healing—direct communication with patients?" [3]

—M.C. Livingston

The following "new" Hippocratic Oath was written by a 1987 University of Minnesota medical school graduate, and has since been used by the school as a teaching tool:

In the tradition of Hippocrates and the men and women through the ages who have dedicated their lives to the art and science of medicine I make the following pledge:

The respect, dignity of patients, and the confidential nature of our relationship is foremost in my service to them. I will value their lives as I value my own.

I acknowledge my limitations and need for continued education. I will seek the knowledge and inspiration of my colleagues, friends and patients.

My work shall be dedicated to improving the quality of life for those who seek my assistance. I will honor the wishes and needs of the patient, recognizing that death is not always an enemy. I will do no harm.

I will strive always to improve the practice of medicine, to provide a level of care that is ethical, moral, and just. I expect the same standards from my colleagues and will not tolerate their indifference, greed or unethical behavior.

My profession is an honored one. I will not violate the trust society has place in me by allowing religion, race or creed to affect my judgment or ability to take care of patients. I will be humble.

I will consider the tools of my profession to be knowledge, compassion, and patience. I will share these tools freely with my colleagues and patients alike.

I shall do my utmost to provide the vulnerable members of society the care and attention they need to assure their health, dignity, and protection. I see all life as sacred.

In the presence of my teachers, my family, and my friends I make these promises solemnly and freely. With this oath I willingly assume the rewards and responsibilities of a physician.*

11

THE MAKING OF A GOOD PATIENT

The process of questioning authority and demanding answers will, in the long run, strengthen rather than weaken both the patient's relations to his or her doctor and the doctor's own relation to career and profession. [1]

—Peter Gott, M.D.

S OCIETY'S ideas about the patient's role in the doctor-patient relationship are changing. Patients today are asking for explanations concerning treatments and they expect to be involved in decisions regarding their care. I see these as positive steps for both patients and physicians. People feel less helpless when they are involved in their care, and physicians need not shoulder full responsibility for outcomes when the decisions are jointly made.

The patient stands to lose the most if the wrong approach to treatment is chosen and, therefore, should have some choices about risks they want to take. During the latter years of my illness, when my involuntary movement disorder worsened, a Mayo Clinic doctor mentioned the possibility of trying an experimental spinal cord surgery if a series of trial medications failed to help. I was thankful to be cured before we ever discussed this further, but if things hadn't improved I might have considered the surgery. I would have wanted to be informed of all the risks, and I would not have wanted someone else to make the decision about whether or not it should be done.

People often benefit from being actively involved in their care. I could fill another book with stories of patients who have aided in their own diagnoses by doing their own medical research. I'll include just a few examples to illustrate the point.

When Anita Bahl's physician could not explain her extreme fatigue and weakness after several visits, Anita embarked on her own investigation and learned that the thyroid medication she had been taking for several months could deplete potassium levels. Once she brought this possibility to her doctor's attention, a blood test was done, proving that her potassium levels were indeed very low, and her symptoms were easily resolved with potassium supplements.

When Mark LaCanne was diagnosed as having an acoustic neuroma (an uncommon brain tumor), he was referred to a Minnesota surgeon who informed him that his only choice was to have the tumor surgically removed, and there was a 25 percent chance the surgery would leave him paralyzed. Before undergoing the surgery, he and his wife, Therese, talked to other physicians and learned that a group of California surgeons specializing in removing this kind of tumor had a less than three percent failure rate. Needless to say, they decided it was in their best interests to incur the extra personal costs to fly to California for the surgery.

Following back surgery, physician Mary Ezzo was in a great deal of pain and suspected she had developed an infection in the bone as a complication of the surgery. When nodules began popping out just under the skin in her hand and foot, she was convinced the infection had spread to the blood and was then forming collections of bacteria under the skin (known as septic emboli). She consulted an infectious disease specialist for help who immediately refuted her theory, saying she was too young to have this problem (it is usually seen in elderly, debilitated people). Mary then called her partner who assisted her in opening one of the nodules and examining the contents under a microscope. Mary was right. She had a staph infection. When the infectious disease specialist she had seen earlier was called back to insert a central intravenous line to administer antibiotics, he shook his head saying, "I never would have believed it."

If any of these patients had been passive patients, the odds of positive outcomes would have been much lower.

I agree with many of the doctors I interviewed who say the tone of the relationship is usually set by the physician, and the biggest share of the responsibility for developing a good rapport falls on the physician. However, the patient can facilitate the relationship by starting out with realistic expectations. And, while it is appropriate for patients to question decisions and at times be their own medical detectives, a good patient should also be honest with and respectful of doctors whose care they are under.

In some cases, a relationship that starts off on rocky ground can be mended and turned into a constructive one. Bonnie Harrison, a lupus patient, emphasizes the importance of getting to know a doctor before assuming the relationship won't work. She says she was very turned off by the manner of the physician who initially diagnosed her: "He seemed callous and abrupt. In fact, I was not sure I wanted to continue working with this doctor." But after giving the relationship some time, she learned more about the doctor, which made it easier for her to understand his manner:

He had worked for many years in a rough part of the city and frequently dealt with gang members who were rather cynical about life. I suspect that had a lot to do with the way he learned to respond to patients. Also, one day when I questioned him about his feelings, he confided how difficult it is for him to treat people when there is not much that can be done except prescribe medication that might temporarily help the symptoms, but will most likely have terrible side effects in the long run.

Bonnie also says that after she made it clear that she wanted as much information about her condition and treatments as possible, the doctor was very willing to take time to provide that information. She now feels that she and her doctor have an excellent relationship. After listening to people in a lupus support group complain about their problems with doctors, Bonnie feels that too often patients expect their doctors to read their minds, then blame them when the relationship is not working. She adds:

> If you don't ask questions and let your doctor know what your needs are, he probably will assume that you don't want any more information or that you understand better than you really do. It's also very important for patients to be honest with doctors. Since doctors often do encounter patients who are not very honest about things such as alcohol consumption, I think that doctors need to learn to trust you as much as you need to learn to trust them.

Since doctors take an oath, I thought it would be pertinent to come up with an oath for patients to help clarify their role in facilitating a relationship that works in their own best interests. If every patient would start out reaffirming the agenda described in the following Patient Oath, it would help the doctor to establish a relationship based on teamwork.

The Patient Oath

Although I have the right to explanations regarding a doctor's decisions or recommendations, I will not demand that a doctor prescribe tests or treatments that he or she truly does not believe are in my best interests.

I understand that medicine is not a perfect science; I will allow room for inevitable errors and be forgiving when they occur if I sense the doctor is doing his or her best.

I will not ask a doctor to manipulate a diagnosis for economic gain.

As much as I would like to be a priority patient, I accept that there are times when a doctor will need to reschedule or shorten an appointment in order to respond to the needs of someone who is in more dire need.

I will do what I can to take responsibility for managing my own health and staying as well as possible.

If I ask to be involved in the decision making regarding my care, I in turn agree to share responsibility for outcomes.

I will let my doctor know that I appreciate the good care he or she is giving me.

I will expect quality care, but not miracles.

12

THE FUTURE DOCTOR-PATIENT RELATIONSHIP: IS THERE HOPE FOR HEALING?

RECENTLY Fred Hafferty called my attention to a story in the Minneapolis *Star Tribune* about a young family practice doctor who drove 90 miles to have dinner with one of his patients, an 87-year-old woman. Fred pointed out that these kinds of stories tend to pull at one's heart strings, evoking images of the way medicine used to be. Yet, he added, it just isn't practical or feasible for most doctors to become that involved in the lives of their patients in our fast-paced world.

While it is easy to look back with nostalgia on the "good old days" when doctors had time to visit patients in their homes, and provide very personal attention, we can't turn the clock back—and I doubt that many of us would want to if it meant giving up the advancements in technology, even though we sometimes see them as a mixed blessing.

Doctors of colonial days were not faced with the same kinds of pressures. They did not have constantly hectic schedules. They did not have to justify their treatment decisions with insurance companies. They did not have to try to keep up with rapidly changing technology. They did not have to consider so many factors when prescribing treatments. Costs of tests did not play into decisions they made. And patients didn't expect instant cures.

Even in ancient Greece, when medicine was not nearly so complex as it is today, Hippocrates was quoted as saying, "Life is short, the art long, opportunity fleeting, experiment treacherous, judgment difficult." Today, judgment is more difficult and is likely to become increasingly difficult in many ways.

With the cost of health care skyrocketing, people in and outside the medical profession are agreeing there is a need for some revamping of America's health care system. As I finish this final chapter in our book, just what kind of changes will occur remains up for debate, and the future of the American health care system is uncertain. However, one thing is certain. The role of doctors will become more complex as they are called upon not only to cure the ills of the day, but to plan preventive strategies as well. The doctor-patient relationship is likely to be tested further.

According to Ronald D. Franks, M.D., Dean of the University of Minnesota School of Medicine, Duluth, aside from traditional training, future physicians will need training in many additional areas. With a teamwork approach emerging as the norm in many health care settings, they will need training in leadership skills to prepare them to coordinate teams of variously trained health care professionals. Medical students and residents, he says, will also need to learn quality improvement strategies and "more sophisticated approaches to resource allocation" which will involve advanced training in medical ethics and associated decision making. "Available resources will not keep pace with the demand for new technologies as well as routine health care service," he explains. "Thus, physicians will need to know how to make decisions to ensure that these limited services are distributed ethically and fairly to their patients."

Franks also points out that the concept of health care in this country is evolving to mean much more than just the recognition and treatment of disease to include gaining and maintaining health. "Thus, the responsibility of future physicians will extend well beyond just understanding and correcting the physical and emotional disturbances of their patients. Instead, health care will increasingly focus on the prevention of disease, both for individuals and large populations. This will require new approaches and techniques, many of which are yet undiscovered," says Franks.

While accomplishing all of the above, the doctors of tomorrow will be expected to step back in time and try to recapture some of the humaneness inherent to earlier days of medicine.

What will happen to the doctor-patient relationship? I see many signs of hope for a reversal of the negative trend of the past fifty years. I had no trouble finding doctors who were concerned about the issue and doctors who had in fact retained the essence of the "old fashioned" caring style of medicine in their own modern practices even though they can't emulate it in its entirety.

Medical students are starting training with new visions, too. I have talked with many who are acutely aware of the current unrest. They want to change the trend. They want to be seen as caring doctors. Perhaps in the future medical schools will be driven by the demand for caring doctors to look for humane qualities in students. And perhaps those who are accepted will be encouraged to maintain the goal of putting the patient first.

Dr. Savett and his wife, Sue, a social worker, give "Sue and Larry seminars" to premed students. They believe that humane medicine can be taught. "All it really takes is a declaration of values from the start. One must affirm: I'm going to practice in a way that allows time to talk and listen to my patients, and I am going to control the flow of patients that I see so I can keep this promise."

After discouraging medical students from going into family practice, medical schools are now recognizing a need for more primary care physicians.

> *John Witek:* Right now there are too few primary care role models. Doctors in training learn medicine from medical specialists, but there are few general medicine mentors. As family practice has developed as a specialty, physicians in these programs are learning more and more how to deal with the whole patient. Ideally, some of this type of training needs to be included in specialty training programs as well.

Insurance companies, too, are recognizing the benefits of teaching communication skills to physicians. Since a large number of lawsuits involve poor communication, some states are offering lower malpractice premiums for those who are willing to take courses in communication.

Dr. Franks believes that along with a humanistic approach in medical training, there will be a strengthening of the doctor-patient relationship, and he adds, "There will be even greater emphasis on shared decision making between doctor and patient, using a more collaborative model. As a consequence, patients will ideally assume more responsibility for their own health as well."

The goal of all these changes is to preserve the good we have now, and recapture the best elements of the past. There will probably be a need to make some compromises, but if doctors and patients are both willing to strive to understand each other, to work together as a team rather than being adversaries in today's complex medical world, many believe that we can have a powerful medical system in spite of ongoing challenges. As Greg Silvis says, "We can have CAT scans and heart transplants in an adversarial setting, but we can't have the most powerful and humane system the world has ever seen in this kind of setting. The doctor-patient relationship is a human relationship that must be built on trust if it is to be effective."

While talking to professional groups in the past six years, I have often shared some of my personal experiences and have gotten warm responses. Doctors and nurses confide that it has been meaningful to them to hear a real story and have considered bringing other patients into medical training settings to talk about their experiences and how the process could have worked better. It would be wonderful to have more doctors and patients talking to each other, rather than angrily about each other. In the long run, money will be saved, healing enhanced and satisfaction increased. In my own case, if I had found the "right" doctor earlier in my illness, I suspect my medical bills totaling several hundred thousand dollars would have been cut in half (because there would have been fewer repeat tests and fewer doctor visits), and the stress of the illness on me and my family would have been minimized. It is very possible that I would even have been diagnosed several years earlier, since poor communication delayed the testing for Lyme disease for an additional three years. The blood had actually been drawn for it early in 1984; it was sent to a state lab and returned saying no test was yet available in Minnesota. Had I known that, or had John Witek known that, we might have pursued it more aggressively, since he was aware that Lyme disease could cause all of my symptoms, including chorea. Instead we were both informed by the doctor in charge (at the time) who had ordered several tests that my tests had all come back normal. I didn't learn until late 1987 that the test had never been done.

There is much to be gained when doctors and patients work as a team, and much to be lost when they become adversaries. Regardless of what changes take place in our health care system, doctors will no doubt retain a powerful role in our society as they have in most every culture for thousands of years. The unique doctor-patient relationship, complex as it is, will certainly continue to be one of the most intriguing of human relationships.

Appendix

Resources for Patients
and Physicians

FOR PATIENTS:

The Health Resource

It was her own experience with illness that prompted Janice Guthrie to start The Health Resource, a medical information service. A researcher by profession, when her doctor told her she had a rare form of ovarian cancer, her natural response was to head for the library. Through extensive research she learned the treatment her doctor had recommended wasn't very effective in treating her cancer. She sought care from other specialists and today her cancer is in remission.

Realizing that many patients, like her, are not given all the facts about illnesses and treatment options, Janice started a medical information service that provides people with individualized, comprehensive research reports on specific medical conditions. Reports contain worldwide information on the latest treatment options, current research, self-help measures, specialists, and resource organizations. Information in these reports is gleaned by computer from medical school, university, and public libraries. Bound reports range in length from 50 to 250 pages.

The comprehensive reports range from $100 to $250. Many patients verify that the company has provided them invaluable information, helping them to make informed decisions regarding their medical care. The service has also received rave reviews in a number of national health newsletters and magazines. For more information: The Health Resource, Janice R. Guthrie, 564 Locust Street, Conway, Arkansas 72032; call 1-800-949-0090 or 501-329-5272; FAX 501-329-9489.

The Patient's Advocate

This is a national newsletter for people who have undiagnosed medical problems. Published and edited by Linda Hanner, the goal of this publication is to provide encouragement, educate people about the diagnostic process and empower them to make their way through the medical maze. Included in each issue are inspirational personal stories, tips for getting along with doctors, pertinent book reviews, information about diseases that are typically difficult to diagnose, and suggestions for living successfully with an undiagnosed illness and for keeping relationships strong. A one-year subscription (six issues) is $15 from Kashan Publishing, P.O. Box 307, Delano, Minnesota 55328.

FOR PHYSICIANS:

American Academy on Physician and Patient

The American Academy on Physician and Patient (originally the Task Force on Doctor and Patient) was formed 14 years ago by internist Mack Lipkin, Jr., and a group of other internists and medical educators concerned about the deteriorating relationship between doctors and patients. Every year the Academy coordinates a national, five-day course for faculty physicians and full-time practitioners, plus a dozen short seminars at schools and hospitals around the country.

Robert Rowntree, a physician who attended a course presented by the Academy, credits the experience for his change in attitude: "I have learned that anger at the hurdles of practicing medicine can itself become an obstacle when dealing with sick people. I have tried to clarify what each patient expects from me. I am convinced that if I find out what that patient is looking for, and if I let that person know from the outset what I can and cannot do, and if we agree on a plan of treatment, we will be less apt to disappoint each other . . . I have regained a sense of purpose that balances the darker side of practice . . . I have decided I may be in the right profession after all. (Quotes taken from "Reclaiming the Joy of Medicine," an article by Rowntree in *Hippocrates*, February 1993, p. 37.)

For more information about the American Academy on Physician and Patient, call 212-263-8291.

References

Chapter 1

1. Andrew Weil, M.D. *Health and Healing: Understanding Conventional and Alternative Medicine.* Houghton-Mifflin, 1983.

2. Sefra Kobrin Pitzele. *We Are Not Alone: Learning to Live With Chronic Illness,* New York: Workman, 1985: 11.

Chapter 2

1. Sonia L. Nazario. "Medical Science Seeks a Cure for Doctors Suffering from Boorish Manner," *The Wall Street Journal: Marketplace,* March 17, 1992: B1, JB8.

2. John M. Smith, M.D. *Women and Doctors.* The Atlantic Monthly Press, New York, 1992:110.

3. "Practicing More Humane Medicine," *McCalls,* June 1990: 45.

4. Charles B. Inlander, Lowell S. Levin, and Ed Weiner. *Medicine on Trial.* New York: Prentice Hall Press,1988: 24.

5. John Pekkanen, M.D. *Doctors Talk About Themselves.* New York: Delacorte Press, 1988: 67.

6. Edward Shorter. *Bedside Manners,* New York: Simon and Schuster, 1985.

7. Dennis Brindell Fradin. *Medicine: Yesterday, Today, and Tomorrow,* 1989: 55.

8. Ibid.

9. Shorter, plate 19.

10. Inlander, et al.: 41.

11. Ibid.: 37-38.

12. Pitzele:11.

13. Peter Gott, M.D. *No House Calls: Irreverent Notes on the Practice of Medicine.* New York: Poseidon Press, 1986: 119.

14. John Pekkanen, M.D. "When Your Doctor Doesn't Know," *Readers Digest*, November 1992: 113-117.

15. Catherine McKegney, M.D. "Medical Education: A Neglectful and Abusive Family System," *Family Medicine*, November-December 1989, Vol. 21, No. 6: 454-454.

16. Ibid.

Chapter 3

1. Eileen Radzuinas. *Lupus: My Search for a Diagnosis.* Hunter House, Claremont, Calif., 1989: xii.

Chapter 4

1. Jenifer A. Nields, M.D., in foreword to *When You're Sick and Don't Know Why*, Linda Hanner et al., Chronimed (formerly DCI Publishing), Minneapolis, 1991.

2. Anastasia Touifexis. "A Lesson in Compassion," *Time*, Vol. 138, Issue 25, December 23, 1991: 53.

3. Paul J. Donoghue and Mary E. Siegel. *Sick and Tired of Feeling Sick and Tired: Living with Invisible Chronic Illness.* W. W. Norton & Co. New York 1992: 40.

4. Gott: 77.

Chapter 5

1. Barbara Huttman, R.N. *The Patient's Advocate: The Complete Handbook of Patient's Rights.* New York: Penguin 198: 185.

2. John Pekkanen, M.D. "When Your Doctor Doesn't Know," *Readers Digest,* November 1992: 115.

3. "Is Your Doctor Listening?" *Vogue,* August 1988: 238.

4. Carol Orlock. "Doctors and Patients Working Together," *Arthritis Today,* November-December 1994: 27-32.

5. Inlander: 154.

6. Mark Flapan. "On Learning I Had a Chronic Illness," *Orphan Disease Update,* National Organization for Rare Disorders, Spring 1994, Vol. 10, Ed. 3.

7. Radzuinas: 59-63.

Chapter 7

1. Larrian Gillespie, M.D. *You Don't Have to Live with Cystitis! How to Avoid It, What to Do About It.* New York: Avon Books, 1988: 114.

2. Ibid.: 114.

3. "Is Your Doctor Listening?" *Vogue,* August 1988: 238.

Chapter 8

1. Jenny Donovan. "Patient Education and the Consultation: The Importance of Lay Beliefs," Bone and Joint Research Unit, London Hospital Medical College, British Ann. Rheum. Dis. June 1991, 50, supplement 3, 62w: 420.

2. Linda Hanner and John J. Witek, M.D. *When You're Sick and Don't Know Why.* Chronimed (formerly DCI Publishing), Minneapolis, Minn., 1991: 155.

3. "Is Your Doctor Listening?" *Vogue,* Aug. 1988: 238.

Chapter 9

1. "Chronic Fatigue Syndrome: A Modern Medical Mystery," *Newsweek,* Nov. 12, 1990: 62-70.

2. Hanner et al.: 126.

3. N. P. Wray and J. A. Friedland. "The Detection and Correction of House Staff Error in Physical Diagnosis, "*Journal of the American Medical Association,* February 25, 1983: 1035.

Chapter 10

1. "My Favorite Doctor: Ten Readers Tell Why They Are Faithful Fans of their Physicians," *Arthritis Today.* November-December 1993: 47-49.

2. Gott: 17.

3. M. C. Livingston. *The Western Journal of Medicine,* August 1985, Vol. 143, No. 2: 270.

4. Written by Timothy Schacker, revised 1990.

Chapter 11

1. Gott: 13.

BIBLIOGRAPHY

Beeson, P.B. "One Hundred Years of American Internal Medicine," *Annals of Internal Medicine* 105, 1986: 436-444.

Bellet, Paul S., and Michael J. Maloney. "The Importance of Empathy as an Interviewing Skill in Medicine" (editorial), *The Journal of the American Medical Association*, October 2, 1991: 183-184.

Bowen, Robert Sidney. *They Found the Unknown: The Stories of Nine Great Discoveries in the Field of Medical Knowledge.* Macrae Smith, Philadelphia, 1963.

Burda, David. "Quality Study Uses Patient's Perceptions," *Modern Healthcare*, Vol. 19, August 18, 1989: 4.

Carver, C. *Patient Beware.* Scarborough, Ontario; Prentice-Hall Canada, Inc., 1984.

Cohen, Daniel. *The Last 100 Years: Medicine.* M. Evans, New York, 1981.

Cooke, Alistair. *The Patient Has the Floor.* A.A.Knopf, New York, 1986.

Crook, Bette Jean. *Famous Firsts in Medicine.* Putnam, New York, 1974.

DiMatteo, M.R., and R. Hays. "The Significance of Patients' Perceptions of Physician Conduct: A Study of Patient Satisfaction in a Family Practice Center," *Journal of Community Health*, Fall 1980, Vol. 6, No. 1: 18-19.

Donoghue, Paul J., and Mary E. Siegel. *Sick and Tired of Feeling Sick and Tired.* W. W. Norton & Company, New York, 1992.

Donovan, Jenny. "Patient Education and the Consultation: The Importance of Lay Beliefs," Bone and Joint Research Unit, London Hospital Medical College, British Ann. Rheum. Dis. June 1991, 50, supplement 3, 62w: 420.

"Drug Addiction Casts a Growing Shadow Over M.D.s," *Medical Economics*, November II, 1985: 263.

Egerton, John R. "Why I Let Patients Tell Me What Treatment They Need," *Medical Economics*, January 22, 1990: 123-125.

"Fallible Doctors," *The Economist*, December 17, 1988, 309: 19-21.

Flapan, Mark. "On Learning I Had a Chronic Illness," *Orphan Disease Update Supplement*, National Organization for Rare Disorders, Vol. 11, Ed. 3, Spring 1994.

Fradin, Dennis Brindell. Medicine: Yesterday, Today, and Tomorrow. 1989.

Freese, A. S. *Managing Your Doctor.* New York: Stein and Day, 1975.

Goldblatt, Ann Dudley. "A Warning for Physicians: A Decline in Trust," *Current*, February, 1990: 4.

Goleman, D. "State Hospital Accused of Wrong Diagnoses, Fueling Debate Over Nation's Mental Care," *New York Times*, April 23, 1985: C8.

Gott, Peter, M.D. *No House Calls: Irreverent Notes on the Practice of Medicine.* New York: Poseidon Press, 1986.

Hanner, Linda, and John J. Witek, M.D. *When You're Sick and Know Why: Coping With Your Undiagnosed Illness.* Minneapolis: DCI Publishing, 1991.

Hafferty, Frederick. *Into the Valley: Death and Socialization of Medical Students.* New Haven, Conn.: Yale Univ. Press, 1991.

Hilfaker, David, M.D. *Healing the Wounds: A Physician Looks at His Work.* New York: Pantheon Books, 1985.

Horowitz, Lawrence C. *Taking Charge of Your Medical Fate.* New York: Random House, 1988.

"How Your Patients Feel About You" (patient attitude survey), *Medical Economics*, April 23, 1990: 49.

Inlander, Charles B.; Lowell S. Levin and Ed Weiner. *Medicine on Trial.* New York: Prentice Hall Press, 1988.

"Is Your Doctor Listening?" *Vogue*, August 1988: 238.

Katz, Jay, M.D. *The Silent World of Doctor and Patient.* New York, The Free Press, 1984.

Kolata, Gina. "Wariness Is Replacing Trust Between Healer and Patient," *New York Times*, February 20, 1990, Vol. 139, Issue 48152: A-1.

Jensen, Joyce. "Consumers Are More Willing Than Ever to Switch Doctors," *Modern Healthcare*, Vol. 19, November 24, 1989: 34.

Lander, L. *Defective Medicine.* New York: Farrar, Straus, Giroux, 1978.

Laster, Leonard. "Let's Never Forget the Personal Touch With Patients; Remembrances of a Residency Past" (column), *American Medical News*, Vol. 35, March 16, 1992: 42.

Lesser, Gershon M. "Don't Lose Sight of the Human Factor in Patient Care," *American Medical News*, August 25, 1989: 26-28.

Livingston, M.C. "Some Facets of Alternative Medicine— Today and Yesterday," *The Western Journal of Medicine*, August 1985, Vol. 143, No. 2: 270.

Maynard, Douglas W. "Interaction and Asymmetry in Clinical Discourse," The University of Chicago.,AJS Vol. 97, No, 2, September 1991.

"McCallmanack: Practicing More Humane Medicine," McCalls, June 1990: 45.

McCoy, Kathy. "How to Talk to Your Doctor," *Seventeen*, June 1989: 126-128.

McKegney, Catherine, M.D. "Medical Education: A Neglectful and Abusive Family System," *Family Medicine*, November-December 1989, Vol. 21, No.6: 452-457.

Nazario, Sonia L. "Medical Science Seeks a Cure for Doctors Suffering from Boorish Manner," The Wall Street Journal: Marketplace, March 17, 1992: B1, B8.

O'Donnell, Walter E., M.D. "Don't Let Your Patient's Expectations Get Out of Hand," *Medical Economics*, Vol. 69, May 4, 1992: 184.

————. "One Word Can be your Key to Patient Communication," *Medical Economics*, Vol. 69, February, 3, 1992: 153.

Orlock, Carol. "Doctors and Patients Working Together," *Arthritis Today*, November-December, 1994: 27-32.

Paulson, Gordon S. "Words and Actions that Frighten Patients," *Medical Economics*, Vol. 68, June 4, 1991: 134-137.

Pekkanen, John, M.D. *Doctors Talk About Themselves.* New York, Delacorte Press, 1988.

————. "When Your Doctor Doesn't Know," *Reader's Digest*, November 1992.

Pitzele, Sefra. *We Are Not Alone: Learning to Live with Chronic Illness.* New York: Workman, 1985.

President's Commission for the Study of Ethical Problems in Medicine and Biomedical and Behavioral Research. "Making Health Care Decisions: A Report on the Ethical and Legal Implications of Informed Consent in the Patient-Practitioner Relationship," Washington D.C.: United States Government Printing Office, 1982: 42.

Preston, T. *The Clay Pedestal: A Re-examination of the Doctor-Patient Relationship.* Seattle: Madrona Press, 1981.

Presswell, Nanette, and John Stranton. "Does the Doctor Listen?" *The Medical Journal of Australia*, Vol. 156, February 3, 1992: 189-191.

Radzuinas, Eileen. *Lupus: My Search for a Diagnosis.* Claremont, CA: Hunter House, 1989.

Register, Cheri. *Living with Chronic Illness: Days of Patience and Passion.* New York: Free Press, 1987.

Robinson, Donald B. *The Miracle Finders: The Stories Behind the Most Important Breakthroughs of Modern Medicine.* McKay, New York.,1976.

Scialli, Anthony R. "Winning Over a Patient Who Balks at Your Treatment," *Medical Economics*, September 18, 1989: 147-150.

Scully, Thomas J. *Playing God: The New World of Medical Choices.* New York: Simon and Schuster, 1987.

Seligmann, Jean, with Andrew Murr, Debra Rosenberg and Todd Barrett. "Making TLC a Requirement," *Newsweek*, August 12, 1991: 56-57.

Semmes, Clovis E. "Developing Trust: Patient-Practitioner Encounters in Natural Health Care," *Journal of Contemporary Ethnography*, Vol. 19, January 1991: 450-471.

Shahady, Edward J. "Personal-Professional Relationships: Difficult Patients: Uncovering the Real Problems of 'Crocks' and 'Gomers,'" *Consultant*, Vol. 30, October 1990: 49-56.

Shapiro, Howard, M.D. "What is Empathy and Can It Be Taught?" *Annals of Internal Medicine*, Vol. 116, No. 10, May 15, 1992: 843-846.

Shorter, Edward. *Bedside Manners.* New York: Simon and Schuster, 1985.

————. *Doctors and Their Patients: A Social History.* New Brunswick, NJ: Transaction Publishers, 1991.

Siegal, Bernie S., M.D. *Peace, Love & Healing.* New York: Harper & Row, 1989.

Smith, John M., M.D. *Women and Doctors.* The Atlantic Monthly Press, New York, 1992.

Starr, Paul. *Social Transformation of American Medicine.* New York, Basic Books,1982.

Sutherland, H. J.; G. A. Lockwood, S. Minkin; D. L. Tritchler; J. E. Till and H. A. Llewellyn-Thomas. "Measuring Satisfaction with Health Care: A Comparison of Single with Paired Rating Strategies," *Soc. Sci. Med.* 28: 53-58.

Touifexis, Anastasia. "A Lesson in Compassion," *Time*, Vol. 138, Issue 25, December 23, 1991: 53.

Wassersu, Joseph D. "An Ex-Salesman Tells How to Win Over Difficult Patients" (column), *American Medical News*, Vol. 35, July 27, 1992: 57.

Watkins, T. "Physicians: A Higher Risk Group," *Medical Tribune*, June 19, 1985: 16.

Weil, Andrew, M.D. *Health and Healing: Understanding Conventional and Alternative Medicine.* Houghton-Mifflin, 1983.

Wray, N. P., and J. A. Friedland, *Journal of the American Medical Association*, February 25, 1983: 1035.

Recommended Reading

Donoghue, Paul J. and Mary E. Siegel. *Sick and Tired of Feeling Sick and Tired*. W. W. Norton & Company, New York, 1992.

Hanner, Linda and John J. Witek. *When You're Sick and Know Why: Coping With Your Undiagnosed Illness*. Minneapolis: DCI Publishing, 1991.

Hanner, Linda. *Lyme Disease: My Search for a Diagnosis*. Kashan Publishing, Maple Plain, Minn., 1989.

Hilfaker, David, M.D. *Healing the Wounds: A Physician Looks at His Work*. New York: Pantheon Books, 1985.

Katz, Jay, M.D. *The Silent World of Doctor and Patient*. New York, The Free Press, 1984.

Pitzele, Sefra. *We Are Not Alone: Learning to Live with Chronic Illness*. New York: Workman, 1985.

Weil, Andrew, M.D. *Health and Healing: Understanding Conventional and Alternative Medicine*. Houghton-Mifflin, 1983.

INDEX

F

H

I